Sex Kama Sutra

The Essential Guide to Having Sex With Your Partner and Keeping Him Satisfied With You, Learning to Flirt, All Sex Positions, Anal Sex and Much More

Anne Cristal

Table of Contents

Chapter 3: How To Be Self-Confident 43

Chapter 4: The Kama Sutra And Love...........53

Chapter 5: Sex Positions from the Kama Sutra

Chapter 6: More from the Kama Sutra 95

Introduction

In this book, we will delve into something called The Kama Sutra. This book will delve deeply into everything included in this ancient book, including specific sex positions and techniques you can try with your partner! This book will help you make your sex life more advanced than ever before.

If you have felt like intimacy and lust is fading from your relationship, this book is for you! Upon finishing this book, you will have all the tools you need to take what you have learned and introduce it into your life to reinvigorate your relationship. After reading this book, I hope you are taking away some new techniques and expectations for your long-term relationship and your relationship with your partner.

We must approach romantic relationships with a willingness to learn and grow for our entire lives, as none of us reach a point where there is nothing more for us to learn.

Who This Book Is For

- o People who want to learn to improve themselves
- o People who want to be great lovers
- o People who want to learn how to flirt
- o People who want to learn new sex positions

o   and so much more.

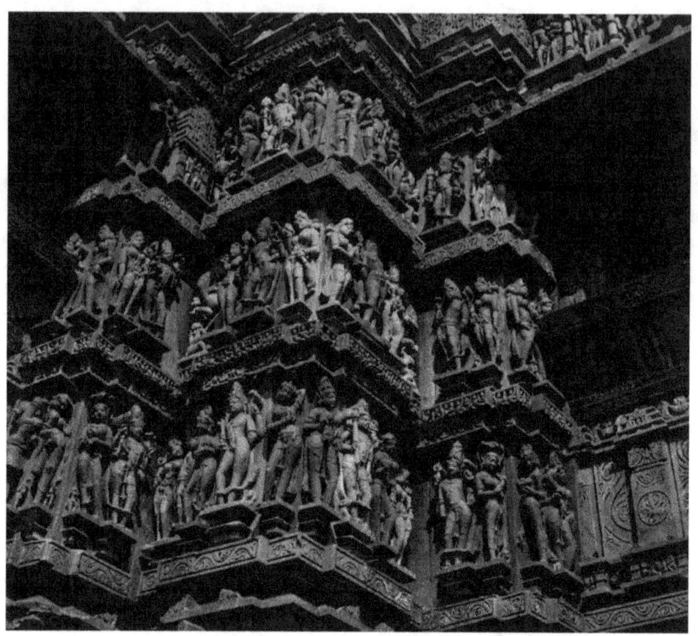

What You Will Learn In This Book

I will begin by explaining what the Kama Sutra is, and I will share some ways to incorporate it into your own sex life. I will share many other benefits of the Kama Sutra, like how to increase intimacy, how to kiss and caress your partner, how to engage in rough sex and how a man can please a woman. After reading through this book, you will have a much deeper understanding of what the Kama Sutra can teach you about sex and love, and you will better understand the history of this guide. The main focus here is to share strategies for maintaining a deep emotional connection with your long-term partner and accomplishing this through sex. Contained here are tips and suggestions on exactly how to continue to have an intimate and loving marriage for years and years from the perspective of the Kama Sutra.

If you like this book, please leave a review on Amazon so that others can discover and benefit from this book just like you!

Finally, congratulations on choosing this book, and thank you for doing so! There are plenty of books on this subject on the market; thanks again for choosing this one! I made every effort to ensure it is full of as much useful information as possible; please enjoy! If you find this book useful in any way, a review on Amazon is always appreciated!

Chapter 1: The Kama Sutra

We will begin this book by first learning a little bit about what exactly the Kama Sutra is. Then, we will learn a brief history of the Kama Sutra before delving into the rest of the topics in this book. This chapter will provide you with an excellent foundation on which to build!

What Is The Kama Sutra?

Firstly, what is Kama Sutra? When we say the term *Kama Sutra*, it is actually about an ancient book. You may not have been aware of this fact, as most of the time, we talk about Kama Sutra as a sex type. While this book guides you through sex by teaching you sex positions, it is a guide rather than a sex style.

You could say that the Kama Sutra is a guide to love and a guide to enjoying a pleasant life with your partner. You can look at this book to guide a long-lasting marriage that will help you keep sex interesting. It will do this by showing you how to benefit from new forms of intimacy.

Most often, we talk about the Kama Sutra in terms of wild and crazy experimental sex positions. There are numerous articles, blogs, and magazines that talk about the Kama Sutra in this way. However, the truth is the Kama Sutra is a book that contains much more than just this.

You may have heard of Kama Sutra in conversations about sex or in articles that you read online. However, the truth is that it is a sacred book written long ago, which contains a guide for anyone looking to get more out of their relationship and sex life.

A History Of The Kama Sutra

The book *The Kama Sutra* was written in Northern India. Originally, the philosopher who wrote it wrote in the language of *Sanskrit*. Sanskrit is an ancient Indian language. The people who wrote the original texts that gave rise to Buddhism wrote them in this language, which shows you just how much history is involved in the Kama Sutra. This book was written sometime around the second century AD, though nobody can be exactly certain of when.

The Kama Sutra is said to have been written by a man named *Vatsyayana*- who was an ancient Indian philosopher. According to researchers, we cannot confirm if he wrote the entire book singlehandedly, but he significantly contributed to the text.

The word *the Kama* loosely translates to mean *affection, love,* and *desires.* This translation is quite telling, as the book aims to teach the reader about all three of these factors. Affection, love, and desire are all very important for a long-term relationship or a marriage.

The Kama Sutra includes seven different sections or chapters. Each of these sections focuses on a different aspect of pleasure. These aspects of pleasure include both physical pleasure and emotional pleasure. Vatsyayana recognized that in a marriage, both forms of pleasure are equally important.

Only one of those seven sections contain sex positions, and the other six sections talk about a variety of other topics. These six sections each touch on a different category of sexual act or situation in which a couple can achieve a deeper level of intimacy. For example, they are kissing, touching, massaging, and so on.

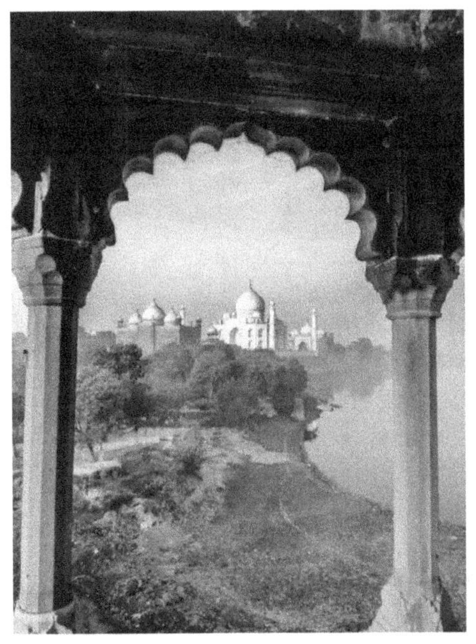

Since he wrote the book in a time and place
surrounded by Hindu culture, it is considered
disrespectful to the culture if a person takes the Kama
Sutra out of context. This point means that you should
not read it one single section at a time; rather, it
should be seen and consumed as a whole. Vatsyayana
meant for people to read it in its entirety, and he
meant for people to read it from beginning to end.
Doing this allows a person to examine it in its entirety
to receive and benefit from the full scope of teachings
that it contains.

What The Kama Sutra Can Teach You

The Kama Sutra is a guidebook for love. This book's pages contain tips and tricks for everything involved in loving and caring for another person.

While the majority of times, the Kama Sutra is discussed about the adventurousness of the sex positions it contains, this is only one small section of the book. The rest of the book contains a guide to many other forms of showing affection that does not include penetration. The Kama Sutra is said to be a guide to love, as it teaches its readers how to love and please their partner in various ways.

Vatsyayana wrote the Kama Sutra with the intention that men would read it. This intention is likely because he wrote it so many years ago. The information that it contains pertains mostly to men who wish to attract and court a female partner. The book teaches men how to treat this woman whom he will eventually call his wife.

The Kama Sutra includes a guide to kissing, foreplay, loving touches, and other ways to achieve intimacy with your partner. These methods include bathing together and giving each other sensual massages- not necessarily the erotic kind.

The Kama Sutra also mentions same-sex relations in terms of one man having multiple women. It also touches on sexual encounters involving multiple men and one woman.

This book is full of information and tips for achieving a close emotional bond with your partner, benefiting any couple. As you can see, this book is much more than a book of wild sex positions.

When it comes to the section on sex positions, The Kama Sutra includes various positions that range in difficulty level. It contains 64 sex positions in total. Later in this book, we will look at several of these sex positions in detail, including how to perform them and what benefits come of them. After reading about these sex positions and how to perform them, you can try to liven up your sex life by trying some of them out for yourself.

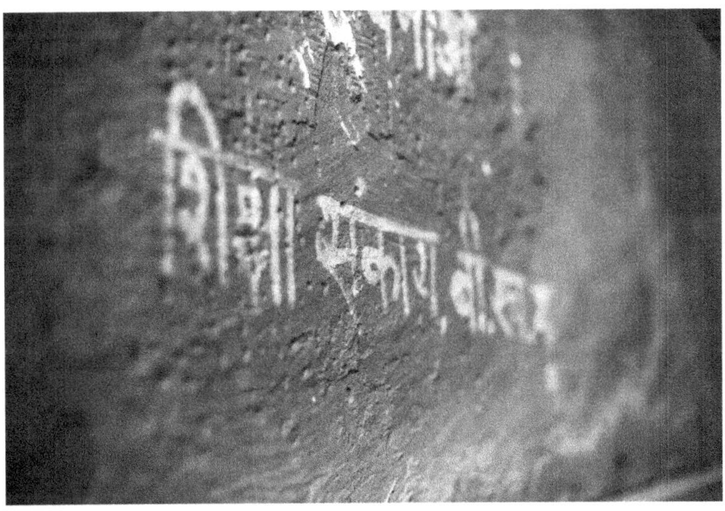

Benefits Of The Kama Sutra

This book is full of information that can help learn more about treating your partner lovingly in ways other than during sex. It can be useful whether or not you wish to learn more about sex positions in particular. It can also help you connect with your partner on a deeper level emotionally.

As your relationship progresses, it is important to keep sex and lust alive. When you become more and more comfortable with someone, the mystery and desire can begin to fade. This fading passion is completely normal, and it happens because the excitement of getting to know a person is no longer there. At the beginning of your relationship, everything you did together was brand new. At the beginning of a relationship, you are eager to have sex with each other because the other person is new and hot and sort of like a novelty.

As you get used to being with your partner, it can be easy to lose those feelings of excitement and settle into the comfortability of your life together. This happening is by no means a bad thing. Getting to this point in your relationship is fun and comforting in its way. This stage of a relationship is different from and, in some ways, better than the early stages.

From a sexual perspective, though, we don't want this stage of your relationship to bring with it the end of exciting sex life. Introducing the concepts and lessons from the Kama Sutra can help you maintain your relationship's lust and intimacy. It can also provide you with new sexual adventures to take on together as an established couple.

The Kama Sutra contains a wealth of information about sex and different sex positions. It includes information about different positions from which to give massages, tips on kissing, and tips for men courting women. There are many sex positions in this book, so there is no shortage of new positions to inspire you if you feel that your sex life is becoming stale. This book can still be found today, even though it was written so long ago, not even in English!

The Kama Sutra's Relevance Today

The Kama Sutra is seen today in popular culture as a kinky and fun book to reference in magazine articles and sex discussions. It is seen as something for the new-age couple to reference for new positions, including acrobatics and flexibility, which will challenge them and is a great place to start when exploring kinky sex for the first time. Kama Sutra does not technically fall into the category of kink, but it is seen this way in mainstream culture. For many people who have never tried anything out of the ordinary (missionary, cowgirl, etc.) in the bedroom, the positions contained in the Kama Sutra are quite a departure from what they are used to, which is why it is considered kinky.

For a book written so long ago, it is still quite relevant in its discussions on ways to achieve intimacy and treat your partner well in a physical sense. You could say that Kamasutra is a guide to love and enjoy a pleasurable life with yourself and another person. It can be seen as a guide to a long-term relationship or a marriage to keep sex interesting and to try new forms of intimacy.

The discussions in the Kama Sutra of same-sex and group-sex relationships are often poorly translated. Translators changed these discussions in many translations of the Kama Sutra to say that it looks down upon these relationships when it simply explores them and mentions them as alternative types of relationships to heterosexual one's monogamous ones, or both. Because of its mention of these types of romantic or sexual relationships, the book can be more relevant today than many other books of its kind. Most ancient sex books, or even more modern ones, focus solely on heterosexual relationships. With the growing acceptance of heterosexual relationships and other types of relationships, this book is more relevant today than many others.

Further, the Kama Sutra focuses on sex for pleasure and not for procreation, which is another area where it differs from most ancient sex books. When this book was written, people talked about sex mainly as something between two married people to continue their bloodline and pass on their status. In this book, however, its talk of pleasure makes it much more relevant to modern relationships and views on sex

than many people think. When people are more sex-
positive and adventurous than ever before, the Kama
Sutra can align with these views to give relevant sex
and relationship guidance even in 2019. Its
discussions of sex come from a perspective of sexual
freedom for the woman, and for its time, this was very
novel, which makes it fitting for today's societies. The
Kama Sutra is supportive and encouraging of the
female orgasm, a new concept even now.

Applications Of The Kama Sutra

- Sex Positions

The Kamasutra includes 64 sex positions, which
require varying levels of difficulty and skill. Later on,
in this book, we will examine these sex positions in
detail to get a sense of what positions are in this
sacred text of love. After reading about these positions
and performing them, this book can help you spice up
your sex life and try new penetrative and non-
penetrative positions with your partner.

- Modern Relationships

Though it is an ancient book, the Kamasutra also
touches on same-sex relations, calling this the *third
nature*. It also touches on group sex and group
relationships. This point means that though he wrote
it so long ago, it has become more relevant over the

years as modern-day relationships have shifted and changed. In some ways, this book has aged well.

- Modern Kinks

There are many different ways that people find sexual satisfaction, some of them through what is called a *kink*. The Kama Sutra touches on rough sex and how it can bring sexual pleasure. As kinks and fetishes have become more widely accepted, this book has begun to show its relevance in this way.

Popularity Of The Kama Sutra

For a book written so long ago, it is still quite relevant in its discussions on achieving intimacy and treating your partner well in the bedroom.

Today in pop culture, the Kama Sutra's 64 sex positions of varying difficulties (from a flexibility and strength standpoint) are often discussed in magazines, television, and movies. Many people wish to try these positions, and they have become quite trendy in mainstream media. The Kama Sutra has become quite common in popular culture in recent times, so you may have practiced one or a few Kama Sutra sex positions without even knowing that that is where they came from. Many variations have come from the original positions in the Kama Sutra, as people have always tried to push the envelope when it comes to sexual intercourse and physical pleasure.

Critiques Of The Kama Sutra

Though this book is still quite relevant today, several critiques have come up regarding the Kama Sutra and its contents, especially in recent years.

This book has received criticism for how *Vatsyayana* wrote it, as it was written from a man's perspective and aimed to tell him how to please a woman. Though this book mentions same-sex relations between two men, this is the extent of other non-heterosexual relationships, which has received some criticism in the past.

The other criticism has come from how this book discusses a man's ability to have multiple female sexual partners at one time. The book mentions that a man can have one wife and several mistresses, which is not popular today.

A heavy debate has occurred about whether we should praise the Kama Sutra for teaching men how to prioritize intimacy and female pleasure or criticize it for putting males in the driver's seat in terms of sex, relationships, and love. Whichever way you view this book, it has many things to teach us. After reading this book, you are free to make your own decisions about which side of this debate you stand on.

In the next chapter, we will discuss intimacy and how the Kama Sutra can teach you how to improve the level of intimacy in your relationship.

Chapter 2: How to be an Excellent Lover

This chapter will learn all about how you and your partner can be better lovers to one another! To discuss this, we will talk about something called intimacy. I will begin by explaining what intimacy is before moving onto some strategies for increasing intimacy and how this will benefit you and your partner in your sex life and your relationship as a whole.

What Is Intimacy?

Intimacy, in a general sense, is defined as mutual openness and vulnerability. There are different ways that intimacy can show up in a relationship, as long as it involves giving and receiving vulnerability.

Emotional Vs. Physical Intimacy

In this section, I will define emotional and physical intimacy before comparing the two in various ways.

Emotional intimacy is the ability to express oneself maturely and openly, which leads to a deep emotional connection between two people. Saying things like "I love you" or "you are very important to me" are examples of this. It is also the ability to respond maturely and openly when someone expresses themselves to you by saying things like "I'm sorry" or "I love you too." We find this type of intimacy in romantic relationships and some friendships or familial relationships.

Physical intimacy is the type of intimacy that most people think of when they hear the term, and it is the kind that we have been addressing the most so far in this book. This kind of intimacy is the type of intimacy that includes physical touch, including sex and all activities related to sex. However, it also involves other non-sexual types of physical contact, such as hugging and kissing.

The Importance Of Intimacy

In a romantic or sexual relationship, intimacy is a given. You would not enter a romantic relationship without some degree of emotional intimacy, and a sexual relationship by definition involves physical intimacy. For a romantic relationship to be successful, both forms of intimacy must be present between the partners. Without intimacy, there is nothing that sets a romantic relationship apart from an everyday friendship. Intimacy is something that any couple must work at and maintain consistently, especially emotional intimacy. In a romantic relationship, however, you must also maintain physical intimacy because this is one way of showing the other person that you feel strongly for them. If intimacy is lacking

or if it fades over time, there are some things that you can do to
revive or rekindle it.

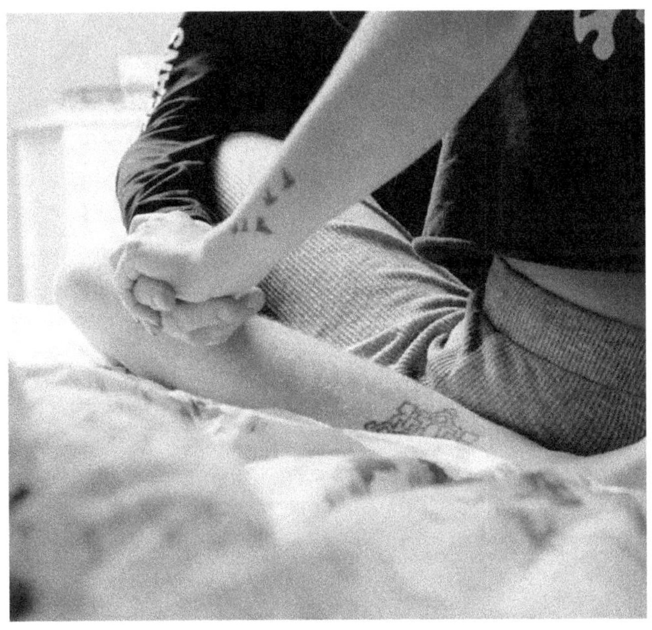

The Kama Sutra Theories Of Love And Intimacy

The Kama Sutra includes many points for loving your partner and how to take care of them in non-sexual ways. These ways include how to give good massages of various parts of the body, including the head and the shoulders, the best positions for cuddling that lead to maximum intimacy, and how you can initiate and carry out foreplay. Because of all of these instructions, you can learn more than just how to have an orgasm, and it focuses on more than just the act of sexual intercourse. This part of the text is beneficial for a relationship because there are so many resources for discovering new sex positions on the internet and print, but not so many resources for having a tender, loving relationship. Reading the Kama Sutra sections concerned with intimacy and foreplay will benefit your relationship in several ways.

Think back on the previous section, where we talked about intimacy and how it can benefit your relationship. To achieve greater intimacy, you can learn techniques and methods in the Kama Sutra that will help you get there.

How To Increase Intimacy

Sex can mean something different to everyone, based on your own experiences and preferences. Sex itself can include a variety of things. Still, in general, it is the act between two physical intimacy people, including the vagina, the penis, the mouth, the anus, the breasts, the hands, and the body. These bodies come together to create pleasure for one another and sometimes to create another human entirely. What you consider sex may be different from someone else's definition, but all sex is sex as long as there are consent and respect.

There are some ways that you can maintain a good
level of emotional intimacy with your partner, to
ensure that you remain connected and in love for as
long as possible. Below, I have outlined some of these
ways.

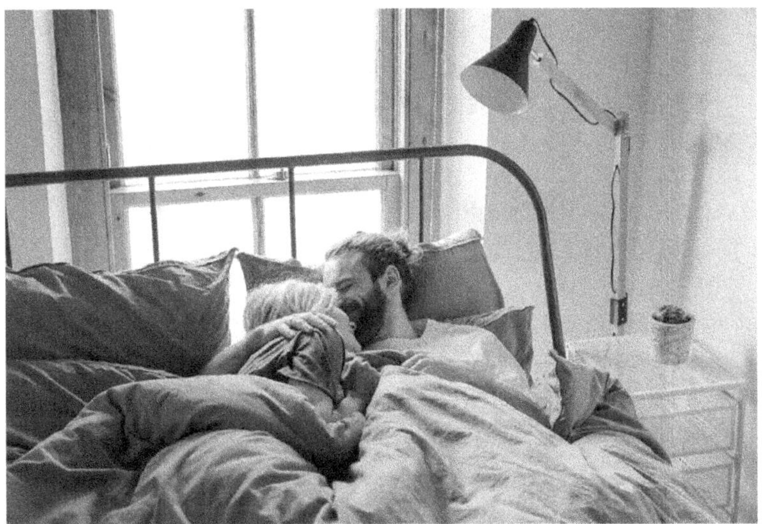

Communicate

The first way to restore intimacy in a relationship or
to develop it in the first place is through
communication. Communication is key in a
relationship of any sort, but especially in a romantic
relationship. Communicating is the only sure way to
know where the other person stands regarding their
thoughts and feelings. Being able to be vulnerable and
open with your emotions is a requirement for
intimacy. It is necessary to share oneself with the

other person in a relationship. This mutual sharing of yourselves will lead to intimacy in the first place or an increase in intimacy.

It is important to regularly communicate about your needs for intimacy since people will grow and change throughout a relationship. Especially in a long-term relationship, being aware of when a person's intimacy needs change is important to maintaining a good intimacy level.

When working on intimacy, it helps to start slowly by talking about easier things for you to open up about- like your future goals or your ideal job. This way is still a way to open up without pushing yourself too far right away. It can be scary to be that vulnerable with someone. It is also helpful to note that there are things that they consciously avoid thinking about, as they may be painful to address for many people. It will be very difficult for them to voice these things to themselves, let alone another person, so allow them to start slowly and not be offended if you feel like there are topics that they are uncomfortable talking about.

Many people have a fear of intimacy, and this is also worth noting. Because intimacy needs trust to develop, it can be hard for some people who have had past experiences that make it hard for them to trust people. Being aware of this may help you understand why your partner has trouble opening up. It may also help you if you have a fear of intimacy as you can explain this to your partner to ask for the patience you will need as you begin to open up and be vulnerable with them.

It is a slow build and not a race to the finish line for improving intimacy. Be patient with yourself and your partner, and try to see intimacy as a growing experience between you that will continue throughout the entire duration of your relationship.

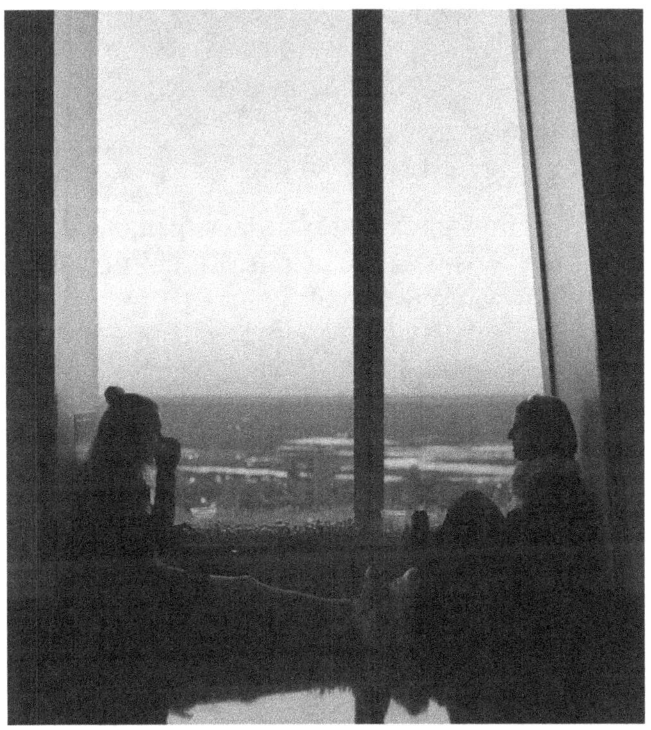

Spend Time

The first way is to spend time with your partner doing things that you find enjoyable, that you can share. When you spend quality time together, even if you are not doing anything extremely exciting, having time to talk and connect simply will help you maintain your connection with each other and continue to understand each other on a deep level as you both change and grow.

Be Curious

This conversation about increasing intimacy brings us to our next point, which is to stay curious. Remaining curious in your relationship is one of the most important things you can do. By remaining curious about your partner and making an effort to get to know them repeatedly, you will keep your relationship interesting, and you will keep knowing your partner even as they may change. It is important to get to know every part of your partner, including their likes and dislikes of food, sex, television shows, and so on.

You also want to remain curious about your relationship. By remaining curious about your relationship, you can consistently ensure that you will be giving your all and making it the best relationship it can be. Remain curious about what you can do better and work well in your relationship with your partner.

Best Sex Positions For Increasing Intimacy

As you now know, intimacy is something that needs to be worked at and practiced. It needs to be actively maintained and does not remain high just because you achieved it once. As a couple, there are many ways to work on your intimacy, and sex is one of those ways. Sex also happens to come with many other benefits. Still, these positions we will explore are included because they are the best for creating intimacy and connection for you and your partner. These sex positions will be great for keeping the intimacy level high in your relationship, no matter how long you have been together.

The Lotus Position

Arguably the most intimate position of them all is The Lotus. The Lotus position is most intimate because of your entire bodies' closeness, infinitely pressed against each other at all points from head to toe, while being face to face.

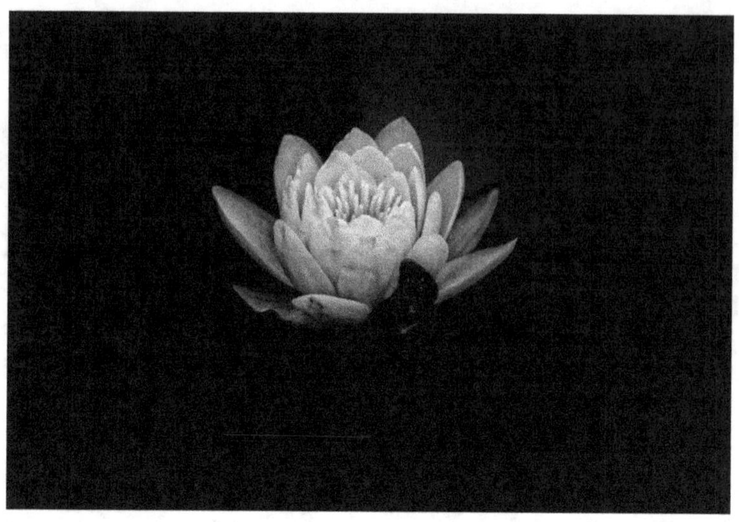

The man sits on the bed cross-legged, his torso upright. His penis is erect and ready to get it on. The woman climbs on top of him and sits in his lap, wrapping her arms and legs around him. He holds her by wrapping his arms around her as well. With some shifting, they slide his penis inside of her. In this position, both people will be grinding more than they will be thrusting or humping. This action is also what makes it so intimate. At the same time, she sits on his lap with him inside of her, grinding face-to-face about as intimate as it gets.

In this position, you will not be doing any crazy thrusting, so it is ideal for a steamy make-out session, as your mouths will be so close that you can feel each other's breath the entire time. You can look into each other's eyes and whisper sweet nothings to them as you share this intimate experience.

Ditto

In this position, the man will sit leaning back in a reclining chair or a bed while leaning against the headboard. The woman will climb on top of him, facing the same way he is facing, and sit on him so that her body is in the same position as his. Then, he can slide his penis into her vagina, and then she will take control. From here, she can grind her hips into him and change the angle of her upper body so that she can control the angle of penetration. She can also control the speed of penetration by adjusting the speed at which her hips are moving. This position is extremely romantic because their faces are right beside each other, and their bodies are making contact at every point. They can whisper in each other's ears or reach up to touch their partner's face since their hands are free.

Face-To-Face Masturbation

Masturbation often happens for those quiet moments of self-care in the bedroom or the bathtub. Have you ever considered, though, that this intimate and quiet moment is one that you can share with your partner? Sharing something as intimate as masturbation can be just the thing to bring you and the person you love even closer together. Face-to-face masturbation is a position that can be done in a few different ways, depending on what you and your partner like. To start:

1. Lie on your side facing each other and look straight into each other's eyes.
2. Get quite close for extra intimacy and maximum intensity, so close that you can feel each other's breath.
3. Begin touching yourself the way you would if you were masturbating alone and watch your partner's face start to show the pleasure they are feeling at the same time.

This position is so romantic because there is no other person you would share an act so intimate with.

The Missionary Position

Missionary position is that classic that you may think you are tired of. It may be the position you began with and stuck to for many years in your early sexual days. It gets a bad reputation as the *vanilla* position that is only for prudes. Missionary, though does not have to be known as the tired old high school position. A missionary position can be very, very hot and intense if you make it so! Here, I will explain how.

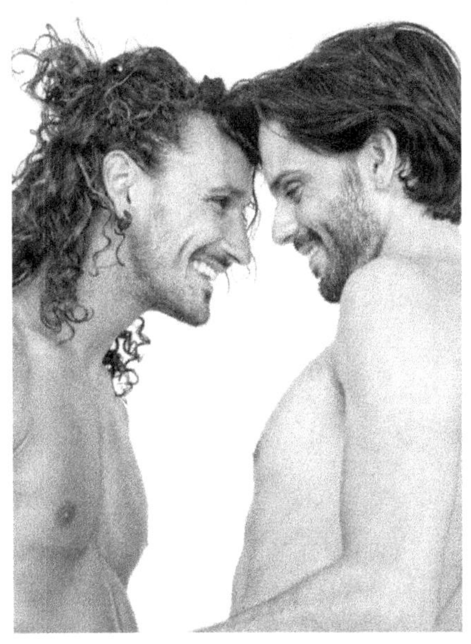

To get into this position, the woman lies down on her back, the man lying on top. His face will be in front of hers. Now, as I said, this position can be very intense if you want it to be. Lying on top of the woman, the man enters her from the front, supporting his weight with his arms. The man controls the movement in and out with his hips. Because the man and woman are face-to-face, this position is quite intimate. You can make out while thrusting in this position; you can look deeply into each other's eyes, wink at them now and then or give a slight flirty smile. When it feels good, let them know by breathing the words "oh yes" into their ear, whisper dirty talk to them, bring your mouth close to their ear so that they can hear your moaning and your uneven breathing in their ear as you are deeply connected down below. Nibble on their earlobe and gently kiss their sensitive neck skin; go in for a deep and emotional kiss. Missionary is as interesting and new as you make it. The woman will wrap her legs around his waist and pull his penis deeper inside of you with each thrust. Your faces' intimacy is so close together as you are vulnerable, which leads to a great connection and a great amount of pleasure.

The Yab-Yum Position

This position comes from Tantric Sex. It is a staple position within Tantric sex and the position that everything related to Tantric sex stems from. Tantric sex is somewhat of a new-age take on the ancient practice of Tantra. Tantra involves being in touch with one's feelings and breath- almost like a meditation. Tantric sex takes this idea and uses it concerning sex. This type of sex focuses on developing a deep connection with yourself and your partner. To do this, you must practice connecting to your inner self and deeper feelings to more easily feel your feelings and reach orgasm quicker and with more intensity. Tantric sex is so useful for couples, especially those who have been together for some time. At the beginning of your relationship, you connect by lust, the exploration of each other, and the excitement. Now, since you know each other so well, it can be hard to reach that same feeling of discovery with them. Tantric sex can help you get there.

To get into the Yab-Yum position, the man sits down cross-legged on the bed. The woman sits on his lap, facing him with her legs wrapped around him. At this point, she can insert his penis into her vagina. This position can be done at the headboard of the bed so that one of you can lean on it for support if need be. Getting together like this brings you close to one another at every point of your body. You connect with your partner from your eyes to your chest to your feet and every point in between. From here, we can begin to connect deeper than ever before. Synchronize your breathing with each other. You can look into each other's eyes if you wish. Sync up your breathing speed and depth and make sure it's not too shallow or too quick. Relax into this with each other and let your feelings guide you. You can do this for some time and let the experience unfold. Try to get in tune with your body's feelings. See if you are receiving anything from the other person in their energy or their breath.

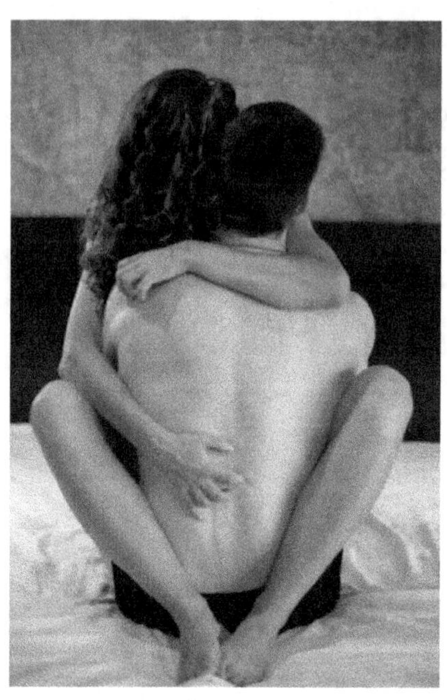

The Slow Grind Position

Another position that makes for a high level of intimacy and closeness is the Slow Grind position. In this position, the man sits down with his legs extended and leans back on his hands. The woman climbs on top of him, facing him, and puts his penis inside of her. she extends her legs past him and leans back on her hands as well. In this position, they cannot move too much without risking the man's penis sliding out of her, so they are restricted to a slow grind. They both slowly grind their hips into each other and move gently. With both of their arms occupied to hold them up, they can only move their hips, making for an intimate mood with no distractions of arms and legs moving about. They are seated facing each other, so they will look at each other in the eyes as they slowly grind and pleasure each other. You can see why this position is such an intimate one for a couple to try together.

Spooning

This position is great for a lovely Sunday morning in bed with your partner when you both have barely woken up and are still feeling turned on from your sexual fantasy dreams of the night before. This position is sensual and romantic as it involves slow grinding of the hips and your heads close together.

The man lies on his side with the woman lying on her side in front of him, both facing forward, the way that you would see two spoons cuddling in your cutlery drawer. This position could easily begin when you are both sleepily spooning in the morning. He slides his penis into her from behind. He begins to thrust into her while grabbing onto her hips. He whispers sweet nothings into her ear and moans. Because he also has an arm free, he could reach around and rub her clitoris while still thrusting away for added pleasure to make this even better. If the woman prefers, she can also rub her clitoris just the way she likes.

Reverse Spoon

Like the position we just talked about, similar but not the same is the Reverse Spoon. If you like the ease and convenience of the spooning position, but you want to look deep into each other's eyes or do a bit of mid-sex making out, this will allow both.

This position is easy to get into the missionary position because his penis will already be inside you. From your face-to-face position, roll onto your side together and continue penetration from this new spot. Both of you will be on your side but facing each other instead of traditional spooning. Here, you can see each other and be face-to-face for more intimacy and sensual eye contact. You can also get into this position from a face-to-face cuddle, but it is a bit more difficult if he has a smaller penis. While on your sides and facing each other in a tight embrace, lift your top leg so he can get in between them and slide his erection into you. This position works best if he is very hard and as engorged as possible, so make sure to have lots of foreplay and dirty talk to have him begging you to let him inside because he can't take it any longer. Once he is in, he can thrust into you, and you can hold each other to get as close as possible. This position is very intimate because your bodies are close together, as close as they can be. If you feel like you just can't get enough of your partner and want all of them touching all of you, this is your position.

The Hound

If you love the feelings you can get and the overall positioning of Doggy Style, but you miss the closeness and intimacy of Missionary, The Hound is a position that you will love.

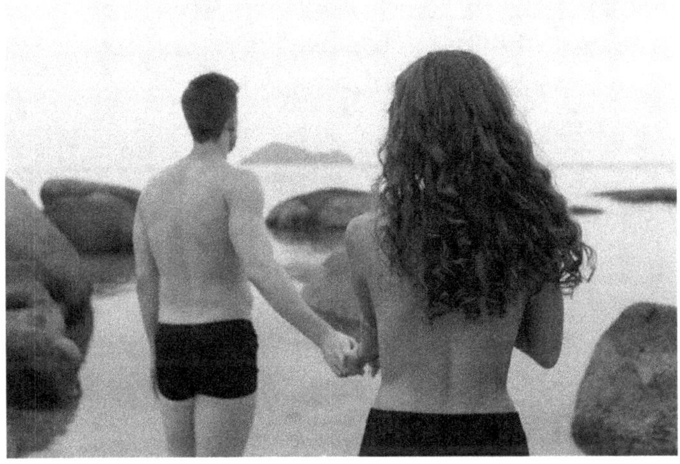

You can transition to this position easily when already having sex in the classic Doggy Style position. While sensually thrusting your penis into your woman from behind her, lean forward and wrap your body around hers. You will do this on your knees. Continue to move your body in the same way, and you will be able to thrust into her more deeply from here. You can thrust quickly or slowly, deeply or shallowly, depending on how much you want to tease your woman and how much you want her to beg you for more. To please her further, reach your arm around her body and caress or stimulate her breasts or nipples. From here, slide your hand down the front of her body and begin to play with her clitoris. Do this while pumping your penis into her all the while.

In this position, you will be able to reach your girl's G spot with your penis, touch her all over with your hands, and still have your face close to hers for cheek kisses, ear whispering, or heavy breathing. This position is the best of both worlds because some see Doggy Style as too distant for intimacy.

Chapter 3: How To Be Self-Confident

This chapter will look at something very important in the bedroom, but you may not have considered it when you picked up this book.

What Is Self-Confidence/ Self-Esteem?

What is the meaning of self-esteem? Self-esteem is a term that we use frequently, but most people don't know the true definition. The dictionary example of self-esteem is "confidence in one's worth or abilities." It is also commonly referred to as self-worth or self-respect. Self-esteem is an essential part of success.

Although self-confidence sounds extremely similar to self-esteem, it is a different thing, though both are important to understand for our purposes. The dictionary definition is "a feeling of trust in one's abilities, qualities, and judgment." Self-confidence is more focused on the way you perform and gives you the confidence to keep going. When you are more confident in your abilities and performances, you tend to be happier due to your successes. When you feel good about your capabilities, the more motivated and inspired, you are to take action and hit your goals. Self-confidence tends to focus on past performances, which then creates momentum to better future performance.

The meaning of self-confidence can be a difficult one to wrap your head around. It is important to understand what self-confidence is before we move on, as we will talk about it consistently throughout this book and in your worksheets. Here are a few examples of what self-confidence means:

• You can value yourself for who you are despite the mistakes you make, the type of work you do, the type of work you don't do.
• You can feel good about yourself and still feel valuable despite imperfections.
• You are brave enough to stand up for yourself. Standing up for yourself includes being assertive.
• You know that you are deserving of other people's respect and friendship.
• You accept and know all of yourself, including both your strengths and weaknesses.

Self-Confidence In The Bedroom

There are many reasons why a person may feel insecure in the bedroom. These reasons could be because of their body image, performance, or ability to please their partner. Below are some ways to deal with these insecurities.

Communication is the key to a fulfilling and pleasurable sex life. Knowing what you and your partner like and dislike allow you to focus on the things you enjoy and leave the things you don't behind. Knowing this will help greatly reduce your anxiety surrounding performance or please tour partner adequately. With so many options for ways to pleasure each other, you don't want to waste time on the things that don't make you scream out in pleasure, and communication is the way!

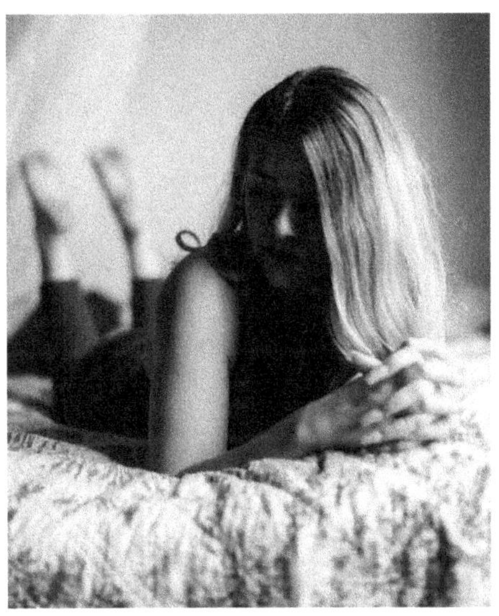

During sex is an important time to check in with your partner to see how they are feeling, what they are liking, and what they want more of. While you are having sex, it is easiest to communicate using dirty talk to not ruin the mood by coming off too serious or too concerned. To properly communicate while also playing into the mood of the moment, you can do so in a sexy way, using sexy language. You should tell each other what you like by saying, "oh yes, I like that" or "I like when you touch me like that" This lets the person know to do more of the same because this is what will get you to orgasm. By being aware of these things and talking about them at the moment, it will help with your confidence in the bedroom and reduce your insecurities.

Strategies For Increasing Self-Confidence In The Bedroom

One of the most effective ways to increase self-confidence in the bedroom is by increasing *sexual intuition*. What exactly is sexual intuition? Sexual intuition is somewhat of an abstract concept, and this is because it is something intangible. You can have all the knowledge of sex positions, sex toys and have lots of experience in bed, but this does not necessarily mean that you possess sexual intuition. Sexual intuition comes from something deeper within.

Sexual intuition can be developed, cultivated, and maintained. It is also something that some people possess naturally. It comes from knowing your body and being in touch with your body on a deeper level than just what goes where. It knows your body in terms of being in touch with your desires, sensations, needs, and preferences. It is also knowing and being able to recognize these things in others. Sexual intuition is also being able to adapt to changes at the moment. These changes could be in your own body, your desires, the body, and desires of your sexual partner, or it could include changes in your preferences and your desires and the preferences and desires of your partner. It knows how they are receiving you and what you are doing and conveying to them what you like and what you want in a sexual sense. Sexual intuition is more than just that, though, as it also knows what to look for in the first place. It knows what to look for in the other person and how to read the answers.

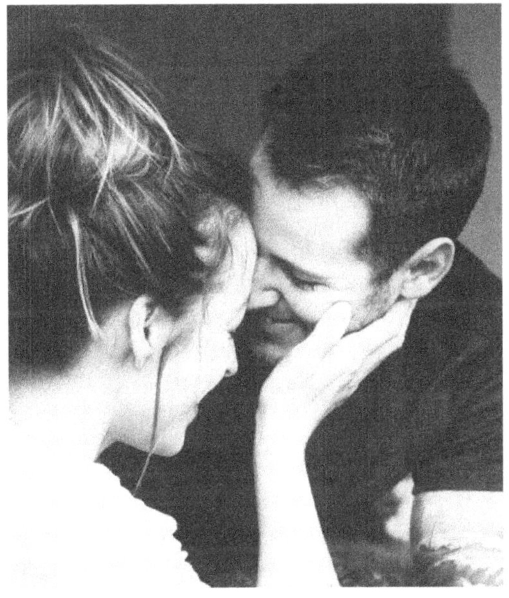

Sexual intuition is all of these things put together. It is more than just knowledge, although that is a piece of it too. It is the ability to look within and at someone else, feel and observe, and adjust accordingly- all of this in a sexual context. Further, it knows that this exists and is something that you want to possess and work on in the first place.

People who do not exhibit sexual intuition may watch porn, become turned on by something they see on screen, and then enter the bedroom with someone wanting to try what they saw acted out. They have not looked within themselves to see if this is something that they truly desire, or if this is something that their body desires or something that will ignite their desires. They have not looked within to see if this is something that their partner would enjoy, enjoying, or interested in.

On the contrary, someone who is sexually intuitive would read about something sexual such as a position or a technique and determine that this is something real that they would like to try. This person would then ask themselves if this is something their body would enjoy the sensations of, if they would like to try this with a partner or alone, and if their partner would have any interest in trying it or only benefit them alone. They then would approach their sexual partner. As they began to introduce this new technique or position, they would examine their partner and determine if they are enjoying it or something better left aside.

To develop sexual intuition, you must put yourself in many different situations and read the situation as best you can. Then, you must communicate verbally. This conversation may seem awkward, but this is the best way to determine your sexual intuition level in the beginning. By communicating with your sexual partner saying something like, "I am sensing that you are ready to have sex?" or "Am I correct to assume that you are enjoying this?" Doing this allows you to determine if your sexual intuition is correct, and if you are reading the situation and the person accurately.

If you find that you do not exhibit as much sexual intuition as you would like, there are ways to improve this. This improvement also comes down to communication. When you are in a sexual situation, you must ask your partner to communicate with you at every stage so that you can learn to match their feelings and thoughts with what you observe. By doing this for some time, you will eventually match what they are doing or their facial expression to the internal thoughts and feelings that you have learned match them.

Just like anything else in life, maintaining a skill takes practice. The way to maintain your sexual intuition is to practice reading people, especially in sexual situations. This practice will help you maintain your sexual intuition "muscles."

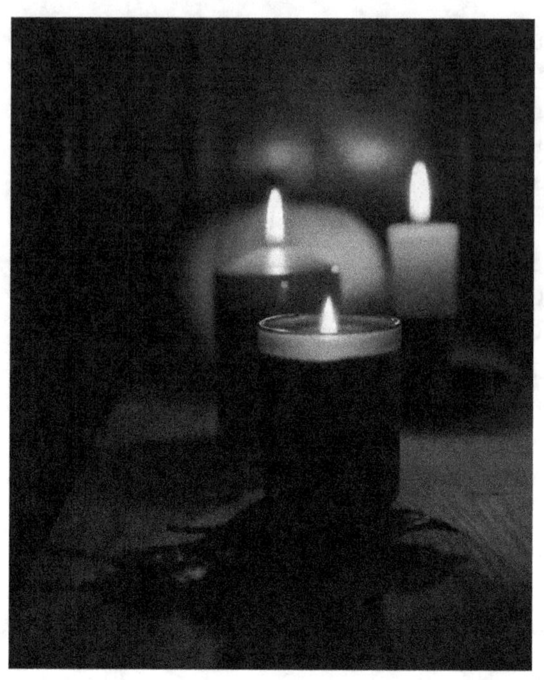

Kama Sutra Techniques For Increasing Self-Confidence In The Bedroom

It is very common for people to have anxiety or lack confidence in the bedroom, especially around things like orgasm and performance. There are some ways that you can reduce your orgasm and performance anxiety in the bedroom.

Your choice of environment can make a big difference when it comes to whether or not you can reach orgasm. If you tend to be someone who has trouble reaching orgasm for whatever reason, these details of the environment, the location, and the time will be important for your experience. They will determine whether or not you will be able to get concentrated enough to orgasm. We will discuss several factors that contribute to your environment is conducive to your pleasure and orgasm. The environment, time, and location are of such importance because being comfortable with all of these factors will allow you to focus on yourself, your pleasure, and your orgasm without distraction.

The ambiance, mood, and lighting must be selected to be simple enough to allow sex to focus while being special enough to evoke a sense of sexy mystery. You can create the environment based on your personal preference, but the main factor to keep in mind is that it is free of distractions and comfortable enough to feel relaxed. This topic leads us to the choice of location. The location choice is important for getting you in the mood and allowing you to stay in the mood. There are some things to keep in mind when selecting a location. You will want to select a location that allows both of you to relax, move around freely, and that will be free of concerns such as cleanliness, temperature, and physical comfortability.

Further, cardiovascular exercise increases blood flow, which in turn increases your positive feelings during sex as well as the sensations your partner will feel on his penis when he slides it into your engorged vagina. Improving your aerobic capacity makes it so that blood will have an easier time flowing to the genitals as your body becomes more efficient at dispersing it.

This effect means positive things for your orgasm as well as your partner's! In terms of sex drive, doing weight training has been shown to increase your sex drive, which is another factor that will positively affect your ability to orgasm. Another one of the countless benefits of exercise on your sex life is that it will make you feel more confident and positive about your body. This feeling, in turn, will make you feel more confident in the bedroom, which will improve your mood, reduce your stress and anxiety, and make it so that you are more likely to reach orgasm.

Chapter 4: The Kama Sutra And Love

This chapter will focus on something that the Kama Sutra discusses, which does not have much to do with sex at all. The Kama Sutra discusses love in a variety of ways, and in this chapter, we are going to look at the theories of love present within the text.

The 4 Types Of Love In The Kama Sutra

The Kama Sutra discusses four different types of love. This theory came about as a result of men who had studied in the humanities and who were interested in developing theories on love and sex. Below, we will look at each of the four types of love.

Love By Perception Of External Objects

The first kind of love that we will look at is love by the perception of external objects. This kind of love is said to be far superior to the other three kinds of love. This kind of love is felt and understood by everyone, as it involves the love for and related to external objects.

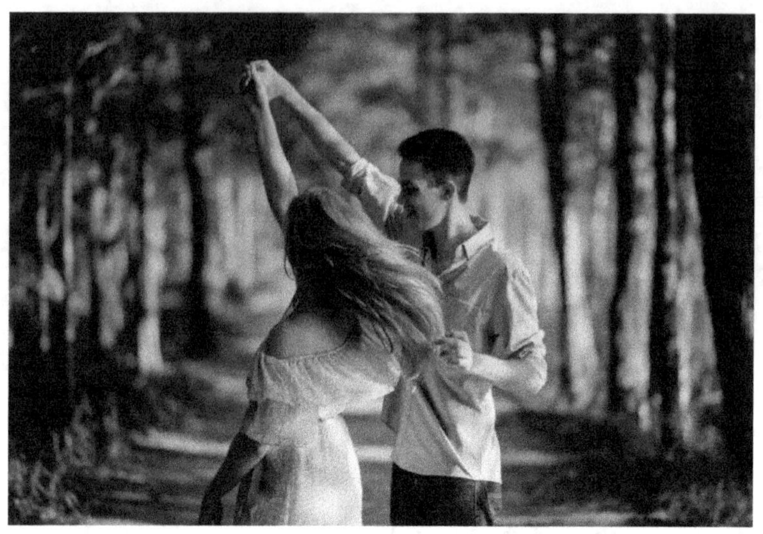

Love By Continual Habit

This type of love comes about by the continual practice of one thing over time.

People tend to spend the most time performing activities that they are deeply interested in. As a result, these activities become habitual. This habit results in love for those activities and the desire to do them often, which further ingrains them as habits.

When building habits, they require hard work initially. Still, over time you'll notice that these tasks and activities don't require as much energy as they used to, especially once the person develops a deep love for that activity. This love demonstrates the magic of building habits, as certain behaviors and activities can become quite regular and repeated, which helps people do what they love and with passion.

What are these activities that people have a love for, and that are continual habits? Below is a list of the activities that the Kama Sutra includes in this type of love;

- Love of sexual intercourse
- Love of hunting
- Love of drinking
- Love of gambling

Love Resulting From Imagination

This kind of love is the opposite of the "Love by Continual Habit," as this type of love results from ideas and thoughts from a person's imagination. These activities are things that the person does not regularly engage in or activities that they have never engaged in, as this kind of love results purely from ideas and imagination. Though they do not practice these activities, they feel love and desire for them. These kinds of activities can include the following;

- Oral Sex
- Group Sex
- Embracing
- Kissing Techniques

- Sexual Positions

Love Resulting From Belief

This kind of love is the one that everyone strives for and the kind that you think of when you hear the word "love." This kind of love is mutual between two people, and they demonstrate it to each other through loving acts and loving words. This kind of love exists between two people who are in a relationship with one another. This relationship is why the name "love resulting from belief," as this kind of love involves the mutual belief and trust that the other person loves them.

The Kama Sutra Techniques For Increasing Passion

There are several techniques outlined in the Kama Sutra that aim to help a couple increase the level of passion between them. This section will look at some of these ways, including kissing techniques and embracing positions.

The Kisses Of The Kama Sutra

One chapter of the Kama Sutra focuses entirely on specific kisses that a couple can use to show their love, get in the mood for sex, or become physical with one another. These kisses all vary slightly, and you can use them all in somewhat different situations.

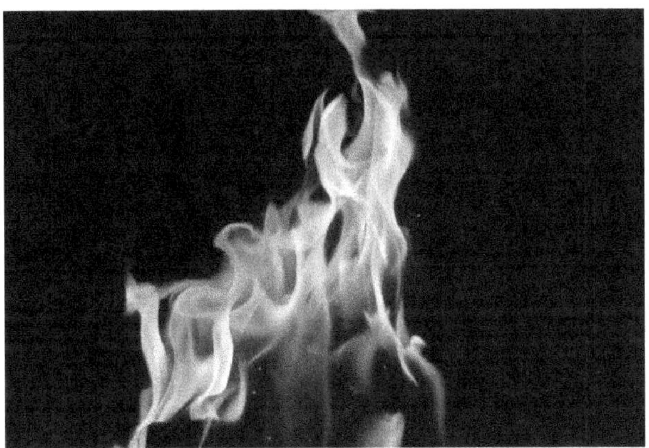

The Kama Sutra states that no set time must pass between the different sexual activities, including embracing, kissing, or intercourse, and no specific order in which you must do them. These kissing techniques can be used during intercourse to increase intimacy and before or after sex. Below, we will look at the different kissing techniques outlined in the Kama Sutra.

Firstly, the Kama Sutra mentions numerous places deemed to be "places for kissing." They are as follows;

- The Forehead
- The Cheeks
- The Eyes
- The Throat

- The Bosom
- The Breasts
- The Lips
- The Interior of the Mouth
- The Joints of the Thighs
- The Arms
- The Navel

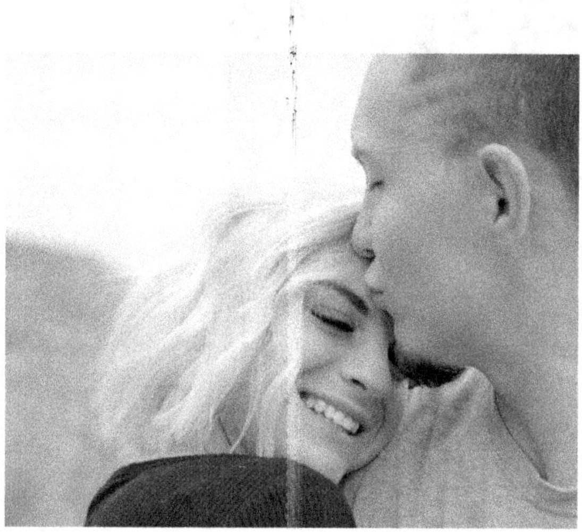

There are also different techniques for kissing. They are listed below.

The Normal/Nominal Kiss

This kiss happens when a young girl kisses her partner with a small peck on the lips.

The Straight Kiss

This kiss happens when two people make contact with their lips.

The Turned Kiss

This kiss happens when one partner holds the head and chin of the other partner and kisses them.

The Throbbing Kiss

This kiss happens when a young girl kisses her partner and moves only her bottom lip.

The Touching Kiss

This kiss happens when the man and woman touch each other's hands, close their eyes, and the girl touches her partner's lips with her tongue.

The Bent Kiss

This kiss happens when the two kissers bend their heads and kiss.

The Pressed Kiss

This kiss happens when one partner kisses the lower lip of the other partner with force.

The Greatly Pressed Kiss

This kiss happens when one partner takes the other's lower lip between two fingers and then touches the lip with their tongue using great force.

Kiss of the Upper Lip

This kiss happens when a man kisses the woman's upper lip, and she kisses his lower lip.

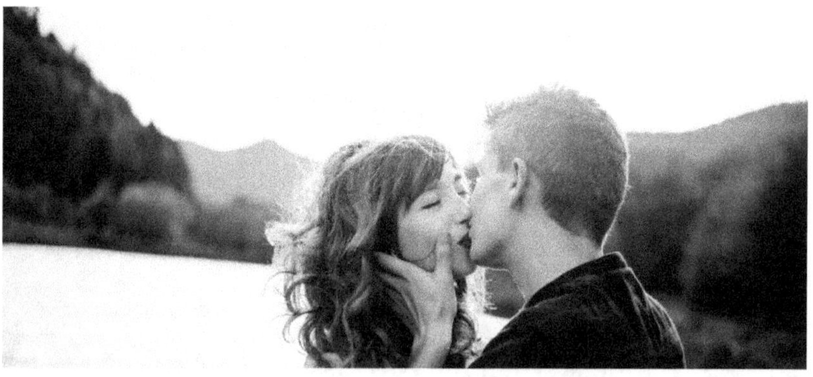

A Clasping Kiss

This kiss happens when one person takes both of the other person's lips with their lips. The Kama Sutra says that a woman should only have this kind of kiss with a man who has no mustache.

The Kiss that Kindles Love

This kiss happens when a woman looks at her partner's face while he sleeps and kisses him.

The Kiss That Turns Away

This kiss happens when a woman kisses a man while fighting with her or is busy with business. This kiss happens when his mind is "turned away."

The Kiss That Awakens

This kiss happens when a man comes home late, and his wife is already asleep; he kisses her.

Kiss Showing The Intention

This kiss happens when a person kisses the reflection of their lover in a mirror or water.

The Transferred Kiss

This kiss happens when a person kisses a child sitting on his lap. This kiss can also occur when a man kisses a picture while his lover is in the room.

The Demonstrative Kiss

This kiss happens when a man kisses a woman's finger if she is standing up, her toe if she is sitting down or while a woman is shampooing her lover's body.

The above kisses will provide you with many new techniques to use with your partner to help you show them your love.

The Embraces Of The Kama Sutra

Another method for increasing passion that the Kama Sutra talks about is by sharing different embraces with your partner.

We are all busy people in this day and age, and sometimes we won't have time to lie around with our partner after sex. How do we maintain a post-sex cuddle intimacy if we have just squeezed in a quickie before breakfast, and the kids will wake up soon? The deeper idea here is the connection and making time for our partner. Spending time after sex is a way of showing each other that despite the busy lives we lead, we are still doing life together and share a bond with them that we don't share with anyone else. There are other ways to show this post-sex if you simply don't have time for a cuddle. However, I would encourage you to try to set aside even two to three minutes after sex. Use this time to get into a close embrace with your partner and just enjoy their presence without distractions of life or the act of sex. To come together without any sort of action and get quiet together. A common practice after sex is that you may also want to share the intimacy of a nap. Any of these cuddling positions previously mentioned will be perfect for a post-sex nap. A cat nap best accompanies the tiredness that you feel after orgasm with your lover. The vulnerability of sleeping naked together is something you don't share with just anyone and is a special moment with the person you love.

These embraces are below.

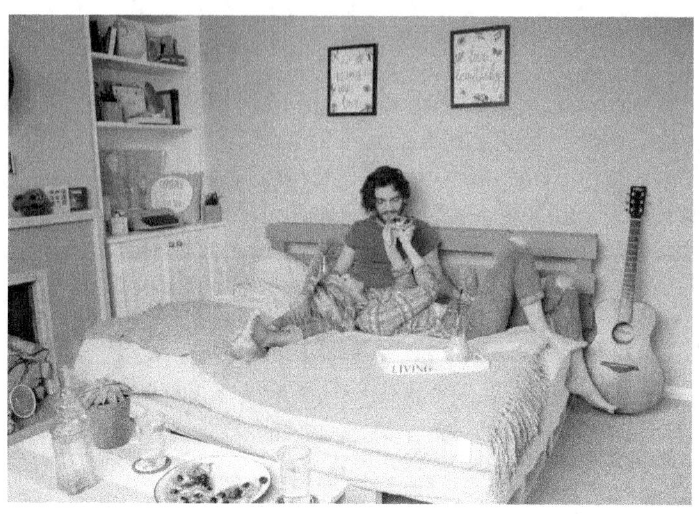

The Milk And Water Embrace (Kshiranirka)

The first embrace we will discuss is called *The Milk and Water Embrace*. This position gets its name from the idea that the two people in this position are enmeshed and become so close that they lose themselves in the other person. Interestingly, this position can be used as a loving embrace after sex or a cuddle before sex.

The man sits on the edge of the bed, his legs planted on the floor. The woman approaches him and climbs into his lap, her face to his. She wraps her legs around his waist and her arms around his neck. He holds onto her by wrapping his arms around her back. The woman presses her body against her man, and this is a great position for cuddling, or she can keep both arms around his neck for a closer embrace.

This position is quite easy to get into and only requires a bit of strength from the man. Both of their bodies support each other in this position, which makes it so intimate. Their bodies are touching at every point from head to toe, and they can breathe together and feel each other's heartbeat. This effect is why this position is said to look like the two people are becoming one, like mixing milk and water when you can't tell where one ends and the other begins.

From here, if they wish to transition in this position to penetrative sex, the woman can position herself so that her legs are open wide and receive his penis. To begin thrusting, they can work together, with the man using his feet on the floor as support. He can move his hips up and down, and the woman can grind her hips on his lap for pleasurable clit stimulation. If she wants, the woman can touch herself during this movement for extra pleasure.

Interestingly, you can use this position as a loving embrace after sex or as a sexual position that adds penetration.

More Kama Sutra Embraces

The Kama Sutra also mentions several positions for cuddling and embracing aside from the Milk and

Water Embrace. You can do these other positions after sex or during a time when you and your partner wish to hold each other and share an intimate moment.

Each time you make love with your partner, it is a bonding experience resulting in increased closeness. Each of these experiences of lovemaking contributes to your shared moments and your intimacy. Because of this, post-sex behavior is very important.

After a great orgasm, you probably collapse on top of each other, short of breath and muscles tired. Having made love, you are probably feeling quite close and romantic with each other since you have made each other feel warm and pleasured like no other. Therefore, after collapsing into each other, you will likely want to be as close as possible. Doing this position lets you get close and romantic with one another for that after-sex recovery cuddle.

The embrace of the BreastsThis embrace happens during intercourse. You do this embrace by having the man presses his chest between the woman's breasts and presses himself into her.

The Embrace of the Forehead

This embrace also happens during intercourse. This embrace is intimate as it involves one partner touching their partner's eyes, mouth, or forehead with their forehead.

The Embrace of the Thighs

This embrace also happens during intercourse. This embrace happens when one person squeezes the thighs of the other person between their thighs.

Jaghana (The Embrace Of The Area Between The Navel And The Thighs)

This embrace also happens during intercourse. This position happens when a man presses his Jaghana to the woman's Jaghana and mounts her. From here, he can practice scratching or biting techniques, as described in another section of the Kama Sutra. This position happens when the woman's hair is *loose* and is flowing about.

Jataveshtitaka

When a woman wraps herself around a man as if he is a tree. Then, he bends his head down to kiss her. At this moment, the woman will make the sound "sut sut."

Tila-Tandulaka

If you want an intimate position, this next position will be best for you. Both overs are lying down and share kisses on the lips and gazes into each other's eyes. Lie on your sides facing each other with your legs intertwined and your faces just inches from each other. From here, they can romantically gaze into their partner's eyes and enjoy the after-sex glow on your partner's face.

Vrikshadhirudhaka

You get into this embrace with the woman putting one of her feet on the man's thigh and the other foot on his foot. She then wraps one of her arms around him and wraps it around his back. She puts her other hand on his shoulder and begins to sing. This embrace is similar to climbing a tree, as the woman appears to be climbing up the man's body, asking for a kiss.

The Head And Chest Embrace

Next is the *head on chest* cuddle. Lie down on your back, your partner lying beside you on their side. Your partner will rest their head on your chest or in the crook of your neck. In this position, you can hold each other with your arms wrapped around their body, and you can give your partner soft forehead kisses.

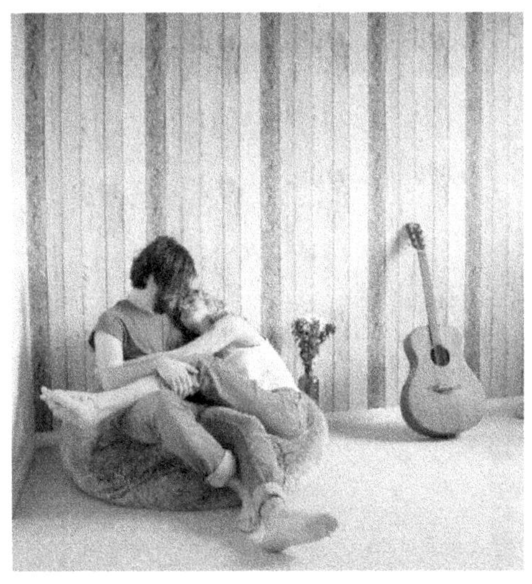

The Spoon Embrace

Next is the spooning position. Both of you will lie on your sides facing the same direction, with your bodies pressed against each other. Spooning is a position in which you can have sex and the man behind the woman. This position is good for a lazy Sunday morning when you are both sleepily horny for each other. If you have just finished having sex in this position, you can nicely transition to cuddling in this same position right after he pulls out of her. When he finishes, he can then wrap his arms around her and kiss her softly on the cheek.

Face To Face

If you want a position that allows you to share kisses on the lips and gazes into each other's eyes, this position will be best for you. Lie on your sides facing each other with your legs intertwined and your faces just inches from each other. From here, you can romantically gaze into their soul and enjoy the after-sex glow on your partner's face.

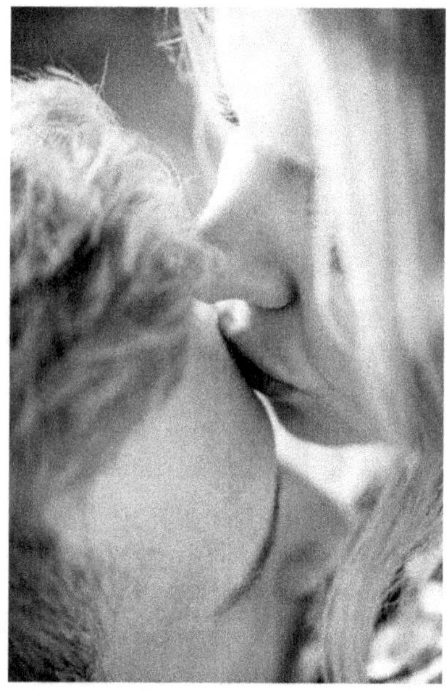

These embraces are perfect for the after-sex whispered conversation that often happens when you have sex in a relationship. You can tell the person that what they just did to you made you feel amazing or that they were so sexy when they did that certain thing. You can share words like "*I love you*" and gentle kisses.

The cuddling positions discussed in this section will help you increase passion and are perfect for the after-sex whispered conversation that often happens when you have sex with a close partner. You can tell the person that what they just did to you made you feel amazing or that they were so sexy when they did that certain thing. You can share words like "*I love you*" and gentle kisses.

Chapter 5: Sex Positions from the Kama Sutra

As you know, the most widely known section of the Kama Sutra is concerned with positions in which to perform sexual intercourse. In this chapter, we will look at a variety of these positions, how to perform them, and some of their benefits. As I mentioned at the beginning of this book, the Kama Sutra includes 64 sex positions, all of which require varying skill and flexibility levels. In the text, some of these positions come with a disclaimer that they will require practice to accomplish, and others are already great for beginners to try. I will split these sex positions up into those that are best for beginners, intermediate, and advanced lovers. As you practice these sex positions, you can proceed from beginner to intermediate to advanced positions.

Before moving on, note that the Kama Sutra discusses sex using the term *Congress*. You will see examples of this below.

The Best Beginner Kama Sutra Sex Positions

We are going to begin this chapter by learning about several positions of the Kama Sutra. These positions are best for those who are beginning to explore new sex positions and increase their flexibility.

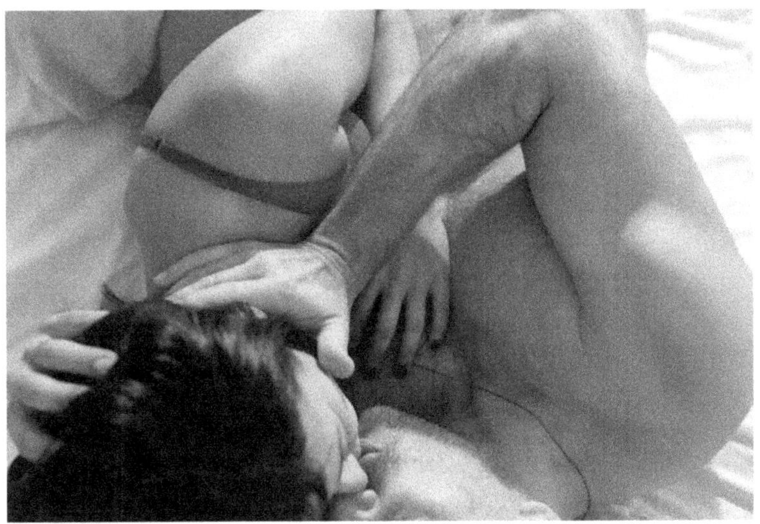

1. The Congress Of A Cow

The *Congress of a Cow* is a position in which the man should act like he is a bull who is engaging in sexual intercourse with a cow. This position involves the woman with her feet and hands on the ground, like an animal with four legs. Then, the man enters her from behind, like a bull mounting a cow. From here, the man can caress and touch the woman's bare back.

2. The Congress Of A Dog Aka. Doggy Style

Like "The *Congress of a Cow*," "The *Congress of a Dog*" is a position in which the man and woman should emulate two animals having sex. In this case, the hare intended to act as a male dog mating with a female dog. This position is similar to the position above, but in this case, it is more similar to the modern *Doggy Style* position.

This position is a favorite among men and women alike. Both women and men can get intense pleasure from this position because the angles at which their genitals come together creates harmonic pleasure for both parties.

To get into position, the woman gets on hands and knees on the bed (couch, floor, this position works anywhere really), and the man kneels behind her. He takes his erect penis and enters her vagina. He starts by slowly sliding it in and gradually begins getting faster and deeper. He does this by thrusting his hips and can control the pace in this way. He grabs onto her hips for a stronger thrust. He pulls her body towards his to get himself deeper into her with each thrust. In this position, he views her entire backside and can see it shake and bounce with each movement, making him hornier and hornier. He can talk dirty to her and grab her butt cheeks from here.

Doggy style is a position that women can get a lot of pleasure from. It is no surprise it is most often the favorite position, especially among young people, of both genders. Because of the man's erect penis curve and the angle at which it enters into the woman's vagina, he can likely stimulate her G-spot with each thrust. This G-spot stimulation means that it will be very likely that she will reach an orgasm from penetration. G spot stimulation can make a woman feel such intense full-body pleasure for quite a long time before the woman reaches orgasm. Hitting her G-spot will continue to feel amazing for both the woman and man until finally, one or both of them cannot wait any longer, and they reach ultimate pleasure.

3. The Broken Flute

This position is one of the more classic Kama Sutra positions. It involves some movement on the woman's part, which gives the man greatly pleasurable sensations on his penis.

In this position, the woman will be lying down on her back, and the man will stand (or kneel, depending on the height comparison) and enter the woman below him. The woman will lift one of her legs and put it on the man's shoulder, and her other leg is draped comfortably to the side of her body. The man can hold the woman's leg to his shoulder as he thrusts in and out of her.

When she is ready, the woman will lower the leg that was lifted to his shoulder, dropping it comfortably to her side, and she will put her other leg to the man's shoulder. She will continue to do this in regular increments. This movement shifts the vagina on the inside, changing the pressures and the feelings that the man will experience on his penis, making the experience very pleasurable for him.

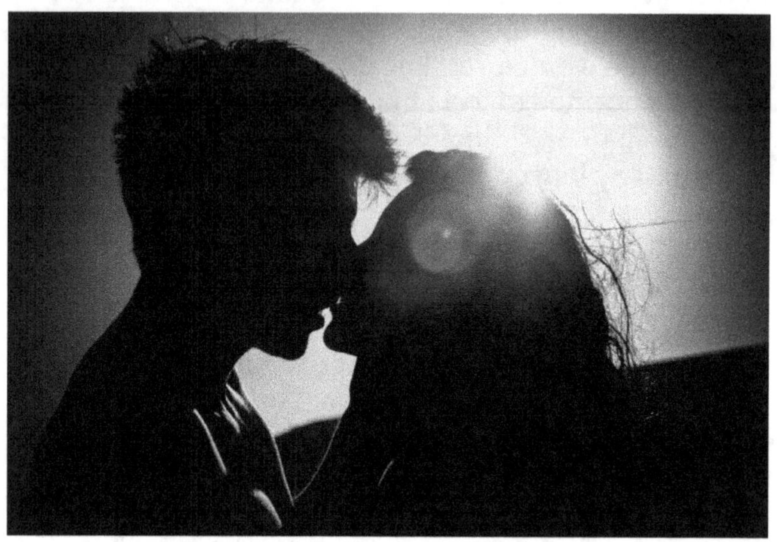

4. The Mare's Position

This position is more dependent on technique than on the position itself, but this could very well change your sexual life for ever. In this position, the man sits, his legs stretched out in front of him and his arms back, supporting his weight on the bed. The woman straddles him, facing away from him, and lowers herself down onto his erect penis. Once inside, the woman uses her vaginal muscles to apply and release pressure on the man's penis, almost as if she is milking it. This technique makes for very pleasurable sensations on both the man's penis and the woman's vagina. This technique creates more stimulation on the man's penis and stronger sensations for the woman's vagina. This technique also strengthens her vaginal muscles, which in time will lead to stronger orgasms for the woman!

5. The Packed Position

This position involves the woman lying on her back, and she will put her thighs on top of each other to constrict her vagina canal and a great pleasure for the man.

6. The Crab Position

In this position, the woman will lie on her back, and she will cross her legs. Then, she will hold her legs to her stomach. The man can assist by holding her legs there, using his body. He will lie on top of her and entering her from the front.

7. The Fixing of a Nail

This position involves the man on top, in a position similar to the Missionary Position, but this is a more difficult variation.

In this position, the woman will place one of her legs on the man's head, and she will stretch out the other below her. The Kama Sutra states that this position will require a lot of practice to accomplish. Once you can do this position, you will benefit from very deep penetration and a high likelihood of G-Spot stimulation for the woman.

The Best Intermediate Kama Sutra Sex Positions

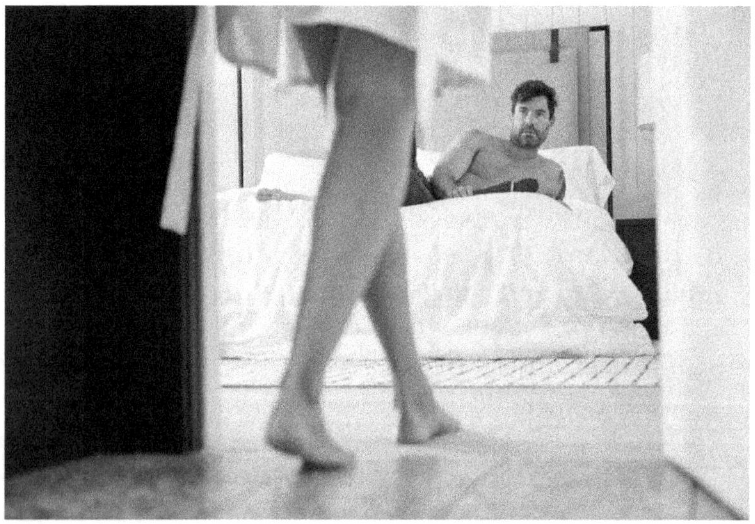

In this section, we will learn about some sex positions that are more intermediate than those above. These positions will require a little more flexibility and strength, but they will come with many benefits in terms of pleasure!

1. The Yawning Position

Have you ever heard of the term 'balls deep'? The Yawning Position creates the deepest possible penetration of any sexual position. In this classic yawning position, the woman puts her legs in the air and spreads her legs with her knees straight, forming a 'V' shape with them. The man kneels in front of her and puts his penis inside her from the front.

This position creates an intense sensation for both partners. This position makes for the deepest possible vaginal penetration of any sexual position. If the woman can manage it, she can slide her legs to the outer edges of the man's shoulders, which will make for maximum depth of penetration as her legs will spread out as far as possible.

There are many variations of the Yawning Position to account for different flexibility levels, but this is the classic Yawning Position.

2. The Lock

To get into this position, the woman will lean back and relax on the bed, getting ready to receive her partner. Her partner will then approach her from the

front. The man will place her legs on his shoulders
and lift her buttocks onto his thighs. He will be sitting
on his legs, which will bend behind him. The woman
will lift her upper body slightly so that she can wrap
her arms around her partner's shoulders or his neck.
The man will support the woman's lower back, and
then he can thrust into her from his sitting position,
and he can use his arms to lift and lower her body
onto his penis.

3. The Position of Indra's Wife

To get into this position, the woman will lie down on
her back, and she will bring her thighs to her sides.
She will bend her knees so that her legs bend at her
sides. This position opens up her entire vaginal area
for intercourse. The man will lie on top of her and
enter her from the front.

This position may take practice due to the flexibility is
requires from the woman, but if she can accomplish
this, it will be greatly pleasurable for her. This
position opens up the woman to receive the man,
which will result in deeper penetration, and thus,
greater pleasure for both of them.

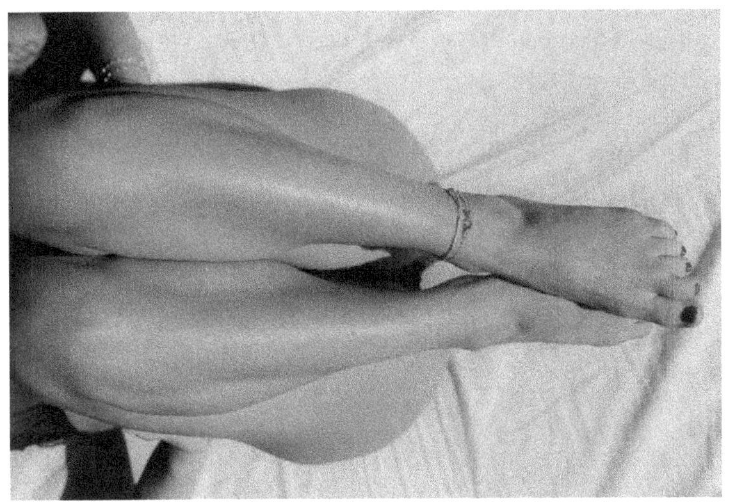

4. The Gaping Position

The woman lies on her back on the bed or floor to get into this position. The woman lifts her legs straight up into the air. The man will then get on his knees and approach her from behind. He will slide his penis into her vagina from behind. The man will then place one of her legs on each of his shoulders. Then, he will lift her buttocks off the bed so that her knees are bent over his shoulders (if their heights allow for it).

This position gives the woman a sensual head rush while the man is penetrating her, which will give her great feelings of pleasure.

5. The Clasping Position Variations

There are two variations of the Clasping Position, depending on which way the couple is lying down. I will outline both of them for you below.
Both of these variations of the clasping position are supposed to constrict the woman's vagina's size, which will result in greater sensation for the man, which means greater pleasure.

6. The Side Clasping Position

You accomplish the side clasping position by having both the man and woman lie on their sides. This position requires the man to lie on his left side and the woman to lie on her right side, as the Kama Sutra specifies. It states that the man should be lying down on his left side in any position involving the couple lying down on their sides.

This lying position involves the couple facing each other, and their legs straight out below them, intertwined in each other.

7. The Supine Clasping Position

The word Supine means to lie down on one's back. In this position, the woman will lie down on her back, with her legs stretched straight out underneath her. This position will constrict her vagina's size, which will result in intense pleasure for the man. The man will lie down on top of the woman, making this position very similar to the missionary position.

The Missionary position is that classic that you may think you are tired of. It may be the position you began with and stuck to for many years in your early sexual days. It gets a bad reputation as the *vanilla* position that is only for prudes. Missionary, though does not have to be known as the tired old high school position. A missionary position can be very hot and intense if you make it so!

Lying on top of the woman, the man slides his erection into the woman from the front. The man will hold his weight up with his arms; he controls the movement in and out with his hips. Because the man and woman are face-to-face, this position is quite intimate. You can make out while thrusting in this position; you can look deeply into each other's eyes, wink at them now and then or give a slight flirty smile.

8. The Half-Pressed Position

The woman lies down on her back with her man kneeling in front of her. She stretches one leg straight out past him, besides his body, and with the other leg, she bends her knee and places her foot on his chest.

From here, he enters her vagina. The woman can move her hips up or down to give varying amounts of pressure to the man's penis for added pleasure for him. Her leg's stretching opens her clitoris up to potentially be stimulated by the base of his penis when he thrusts his hips and penetrates deeply into her. Having one foot planted on his chest keeps her legs open wide with every one of his thrusts to allow deep penetration and clitoral stimulation. Since the woman spreads her legs wide open, it is very pleasurable for both of them.

This position is a midpoint to a more difficult Kama Sutra position, which requires a lot of flexibility. Still, this version is quite good if you are unable to perform the original position.

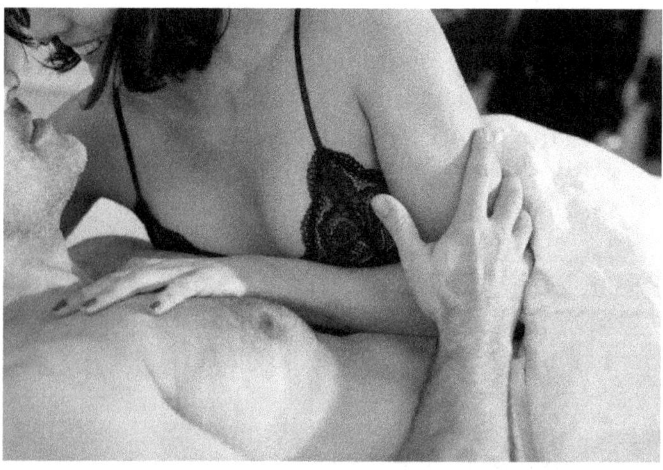

9. The Posture of Splitting Bamboo

The woman will lie on her back, and the man will lie on top of her. He will slide his body in between her legs. The woman will lift one of her legs and put it on one of his shoulders, and the other will stretch out past his body. From here, he pushes his hips forward and can easily slide his penis into her vagina, which is open and in a perfect position for penetration. The man will do the thrusting here. After some time, the woman will switch and put the other leg on his other shoulder. She can continue to alternate as they engage in intercourse.

This position requires flexibility from the woman but gives a deep penetration once accomplished. This position almost rides that line between pleasure and pain due to the stretch.

This position allows for deep penetration and varied pressure on the man's penis, which will be extremely pleasurable for him.

If the woman is feeling flexible and wants to try a new position that will have both of them benefitting from a deeper penetration than most of the classics, this position will be a great choice.

10.   The Supported Congress

To get into this position, the man is standing. He faces
a wall with the woman standing in front of him, facing
him. The woman lifts one knee and wraps her leg
around one of the man's legs. The man can then slide
his penis into her vagina; she raises her leg to allow
deeper penetration and easier access. In standing
positions, it may be more difficult to get the
penetration right away. Still, with some maneuvering
and adjustments because of height differences, you
will eventually get into a comfortable rhythm.

This position is a midway point to another position in
the Kama Sutra called The Suspended Congress,
which we will see below. The original position is quite
difficult for the man, but it can lead to very deep
penetration if achieved. The Supported Congress is a
great place to start if you want to try the Suspended
Congress's full position eventually.

The Best Advanced Kama Sutra Sex Positions

In this final section of this chapter, we will learn about
the advanced sex positions in the Kama Sutra, which
will provide you with high levels of pleasure, but that
will require more from you and your partner by way of
strength, flexibility, and stamina. Let's dive in!

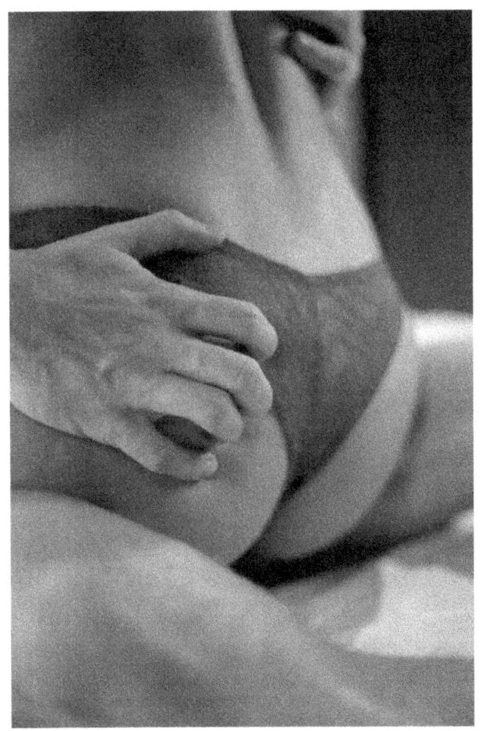

1. The Pressing Position

The pressing position is a variation of the Supine Clasping position. The woman will wrap her legs around the man's body and pull his penis deeper inside of her with each thrust using her thighs.

The intimacy of their faces being so close together leads to a great connection and great pleasure for the couple.

2. The Expanding Position

The *Expanding Position* is a great position for males
who have a larger member, as it allows the woman's
vagina to make room to accommodate his size.

The man and woman will lie on their sides, facing
each other. The woman will lift the leg on top, and the
man will enter her from the front. Once he is inside,
the woman will lower her leg back to its resting
position. From here, he can begin to thrust himself
into her.

Because this position makes room for his size and,
once he is inside, becomes tighter again, this will
result in great pleasure for the man. The feeling of the
woman's vagina closing around him will lead to great
pleasure.

3. The Peg

The Peg has a sexy name that implies pleasure and
may even have you turned on already. This position is
a more difficult position, certainly more difficult to get
yourselves into, but it comes with the reward of a
great all-encompassing orgasm for both parties if you
can do it.

The man lies on his side, and the woman lies on her
side facing him, her head at his feet. The woman will
lift her knees towards her chest, place one of her legs
underneath the man's legs, and have the other on top
of his legs. Essentially, she is hugging his legs with her

entire body. She slides up so that her vulva is next to his penis. When aligned properly, he can penetrate her and achieve depth and control as she is positioned perfectly for his penis to enter her. The woman wraps her arms around his legs, and he can use his hands and arms to help with his thrusting, or if she is comfortable, he can use his hands to stimulate her anal area with his fingers or a toy. The woman is positioned like because it allows her vulva to be open and accessible, which will lead to a stronger orgasm for her. The man being able to see all of her and play with her anus will lead to a stronger orgasm.

4. The Widely Open Position

This position's name means that the woman's entire body is "widely opened" to receive pleasure in her man's form. Her body is in a position that says she is ready for this experience.

The woman will lie down on a bed on her back. The man will lie on top of her, putting both of his legs between hers. Have him hold his weight up, so he hovers you, allowing you to get into position before he comes into you. Proceed to throw your head back so you can see your headboard and arch your back at the same time, pushing your breasts into the air. Use your elbows behind you to support you and lift your hips into the air to meet your man's body hovering over top of you. Hold onto this position and (in whatever sensual language you feel turned on by) invite your man to put his penis into you. While you hold yourself up in this position, he can then thrust his penis in and out with varying speed and force. If it proves to be too difficult for you to hold up your body weight the entire time, ask your man to help you by holding himself up with one arm and by wrapping his other arm under your lower back to support you a bit.

So why hold your body in this difficult position, you ask? This position is great because the woman's raised position allows the man to achieve deep penetration like the vagina is raised and more exposed to the front where the man's penis is. Further, because she presses herself up in an arched-back position, her clitoris is lifted and exposed more than ever, which will allow for the friction of the man's thrusts against her body to stimulate the clitoris with each pump.

5. The Twining Position

The Twining Position is another variation of the Clasping Position, but this is a variation of the Side Clasping Position. In this position, the man and woman will be in the clasping position, and the woman will put one of her thighs across her partner's thigh. This position will allow for deeper penetration.

6. The Fully Pressed Position

This position is a more challenging version of the half-pressed position that we discussed above. This position needs a little bit of flexibility, but it is also a sort of a stretch, so if you ease into it, you should be able to reach it in a few minutes after your body is warmed up.

The woman lies on her back and brings her knees to her chest, wrapping her arms around them, her body forming a small ball shape. The man kneels near her buttocks and enters her vagina from a kneeling position in front of her. Her vagina will be quite easily accessible because her legs she has her legs at her chest. If he has the flexibility, the man can now lean forward with his upper body, and with his chest, he can hold her legs to her chest for her so that her hands are free. With her free hands, she can hold the back of his neck, pull his hair, or caress his face, depending on what direction you want to go with this sexual encounter. The man's penis can very easily meet the woman's G-spot because of its curve, which will make for an intense orgasm for both parties. The restriction of movement paired with their bodies' extreme closeness is sure to make for some pent-up arousal that has no other way to be released than through a full-body orgasm.

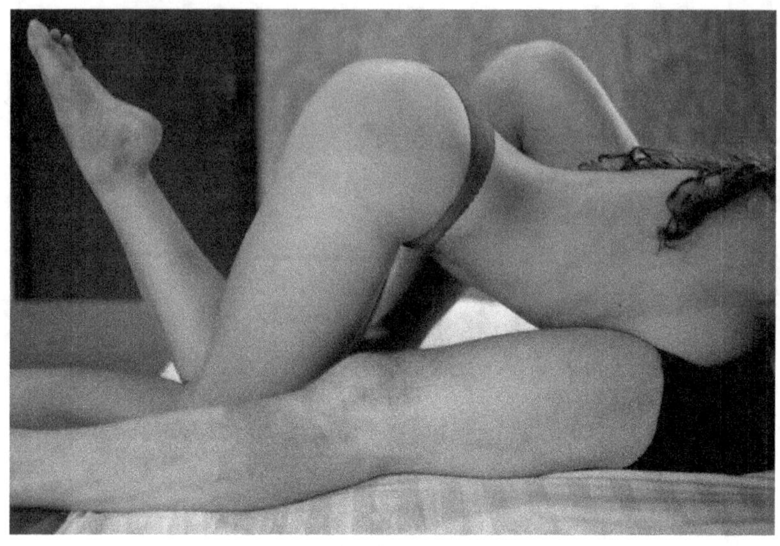

7. The Turning Position

The Turning Position is a fun one that you have probably never heard of before. It can add some fun into your stale sex life or some pizazz into a new and youthful relationship. This position is one of the more challenging positions to master and requires quite a lot of communication from both parties. It will also require some practice to execute it seamlessly but don't be intimidated; you will master it in no time and begin to wow all of your present and/or future partners! This position is well suited to couples who would like to try something different and explore new ways of reaching pleasure together at a point in their relationship when they are comfortable with each other and know how to communicate well.

The position begins in the classic Missionary position (as discussed previously in this book) with the man on top of the woman and both face-to-face. The man's legs should both be between the woman's legs, and his penis is already inside of her. This part is where it gets more complicated, so listen closely. The man now lifts his left leg over the woman's right leg and then proceeds to lift his right leg over her right leg. He does this while keeping his penis inside of her. He then continues by moving his upper body in a clockwise direction until he is at a 90-degree angle to her body, essentially lying across her (while still penetrating her). He will then move his legs over her upper body, one leg at a time, continuing to turn around in a clockwise direction so that his feet are at either side of her head, still maintaining his penis's positioning inside her vagina. From here, he will complete the turn and come back to his starting Missionary position without ever removing his penis from her vagina. Doing this seamlessly and sensually without accidentally pulling out of her will require practice and cooperation from both of them. It looks like he is turning in a slow and smooth circle around her body when he does it well.

This position will lead to new sensations for both partners. These new sensations result from the feeling that every single angle of his penis inside her vagina gives them. It will lead to new challenges for both of them as it is a complex position to try. And it will lead to the exploration of new points of view of the other person's body, all three of these things leading to greater intimacy and closeness between partners.

8. The Suspended Congress

To get into this position, the man will face a wall with the woman standing in front of him, facing him. She will then jump into his arms and wrap both her arms and her legs around him. Once here, he can insert his penis into her vagina while holding onto her buttocks or underneath her knees. He can lean her back on the wall in front of him for support so that he does not have to support her entire weight in his arms. If he holds onto her underneath her knees, this will open her up so that her vagina is easily accessible. The fact that the man holds her suspended, coupled with this, will make it so that deep penetration occurs, which will be pleasurable for both the man and the woman. Deep penetration is great for the female orgasm because there are two places located deep within the vagina that, when stimulated, lead to a very intense orgasm for her. The penis must achieve continuous deep penetration for this to happen, and in this position, it is quite possible.

This position is great for the female orgasm because of the angle that the man's penis enters her vagina. It is also quite pleasurable for the woman because the man is in control in this position, so the woman can relax and enjoy the pleasure he is bringing to her body.

Chapter 6: More from the Kama Sutra

In this chapter, we will look at the Kama Sutra in terms of how it discusses several different kinds of sex that do not include traditional intercourse. The Kama Sutra contains a variety of tips, which are related to other kinds of sex, including tips for group sex and oral sex. We will begin by looking at some Kama Sutra theories of relationships. The Kama Sutra outlines various relationships that we will look at in this chapter.

Before we move on, I would like to remind you that if you like this book, please leave a review on Amazon so that others can discover and benefit from this book just like you!

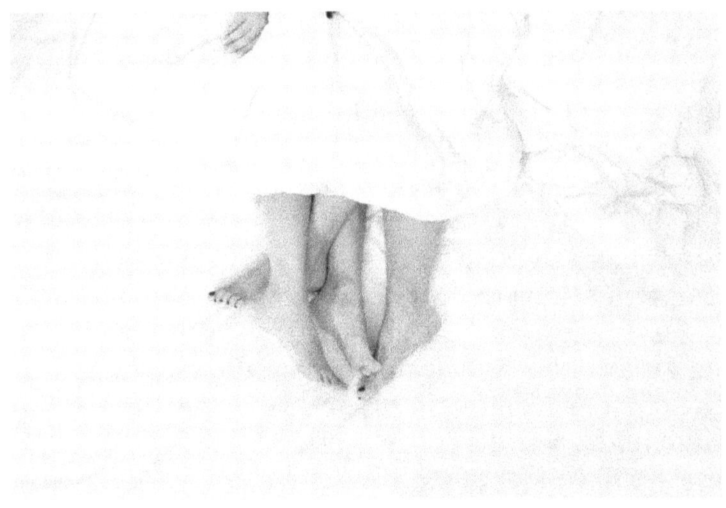

What the Kama Sutra Says About Oral Sex

The term *Oral* means involving the mouth. As you can guess then, oral sex is sex involving the mouth. There are many different colloquial names for oral sex, but they all come down to *oral sex*. We will discuss oral sex techniques and positions for giving oral sex to both men and women in this section, with oral sex techniques and positions that have been taken directly from the Kama Sutra.

The Kama Sutra says that when giving oral sex to a man, her partner's mouth stimulates his erogenous zones like his penis and his testicles. When giving oral sex to a woman, her partner's mouth stimulates her erogenous zones, including her clitoris and labia. Stimulating the clitoris with your tongue is the best way to give oral sex to a woman.

When you see oral sex portrayed in movies and TV, there's only a small handful of easily recognizable positions. That can put a cap on what positions real-world couples think of as options for when they engage in it themselves and can therefore lend itself to the kind of repetitions that create dead bedrooms. Oral sex has as many variants and creative forms as any other kind of sex. By only sticking to the few most common positions, you might discover that you are missing out and a world of pleasures and opportunities to connect with your lover.

Oral Sex Positions

Remember, as I mentioned previously, that the book of Kama Sutra includes various oral sex positions, not only positions for having traditional intercourse. This position is one of those positions.

1. The Standing Oral Sex Position

You do this position when the man is standing up, and the woman is on her knees in front of him, giving him oral sex. You may be thinking that this is not an advanced sex position because you have done it many times, and it is quite common. Here, however, we are going to make it an advanced position.

To make this into an advanced sex position, while the woman is kneeling in front of the man and giving him oral sex, she can use one of her hands to hold onto his testicles and gently massage them. This technique will add to his pleasure quite a bit. She can also (instead) use her other hand to reach around behind him and stimulate his anus with her finger. She can move her finger around the outside of his anus, stimulating the sensitive skin there, and this will make him feel immense amounts of pleasure. Simultaneously doing both of these will make it virtually impossible for him not to orgasm very quickly.

2. The Tee

Like the previous position, this one may seem as if it is common and like you have done it a million times; however, with this position, we will be adding some elements that take it from an easier position to an advanced one.

The woman lies down on her back to get into this position, and the man lies down with his mouth at her clitoris. He will lie with his body perpendicular to hers. This way, their bodies form the letter 'T.' Lying as this makes it so that the woman can have the most pleasure possible from oral sex because it makes it easier for the man to stimulate her clitoris for a longer period without becoming fatigued. It is easier to move your tongue in an up and down motion than in a side to side motion, and when forming a T with their bodies, his tongue can move up and down (side to side on the clitoris) and give her the most pleasure possible. This pleasure happens because stimulating the clitoris in this way is most likely to lead to orgasm. On the contrary, moving over it in a top to bottom motion will not lead to as much pleasure or chance of orgasm. When lying in a classic oral sex position of the man between the woman's legs, it would be hard for him to move his tongue in a side to side motion for a long time as it would become very tired. Still, if he moves his tongue up and down, it will not be as pleasurable for her. For these reasons, this T position is the best choice for oral sex for a woman.

3. The Roll

This position is a wonderful oral sex position. In this position, the man will be stimulating the woman's anus and/or vagina orally while she gives him oral sex at the same time. To get into this position, the woman will lie on the bed on her back. The woman will hold onto her ankles, spreading her legs out to the side as much as possible. The man will come over to the woman, facing her feet, and he will place one of his knees on each side of her head. He will place one of his hands on either side of her hips. He will then lower himself down so that he can stimulate her orally. The woman will pull her ankles toward her head so that her body rolls up into a ball, giving the man more ease of access. She will then take his penis in her mouth and stimulate him orally. This position allows both people to benefit from oral sex at the same time. The man can also use one of his hands to stimulate the woman anally, vaginally, or clitorally while giving her oral.

Anal Sex

As I'm sure you can imagine, the Kama Sutra also has something to say about anal sex. Anal sex is a type of sex that involves penetration or stimulation of the anus. Anal sex includes stimulation of either or both the inside and the outside of the anus. You perform anal sex as a means of achieving sexual pleasure.

Many people enjoy sexual pleasure in the form of anal stimulation, and in this section, we will look at what the Kama Sutra has to say about anal sex and various positions in which you can do this.

We will begin by looking at some things you should keep in mind when engaging in anal sex.

An anal orgasm is a type of orgasm that can be experienced by both women and men. This type of orgasm takes some time to occur, as the anus is a very sensitive part of the body. Still, when done in the right way, an individual can experience a very intense orgasm in various ways, which we will look at throughout this chapter. You can have anal sex using fingers, using your partner's mouth, using a penis, or even using various sex toys.

Heterosexual men maybe a little scared of anal play at first, but this can be extremely pleasurable for them if done in the right way!

Different types of orgasms are possible for men to experience- orgasms that don't involve their penis. This variety of orgasms is one reason why ejaculation does not necessarily signal orgasm.

One of the most sensitive male erogenous zones is the prostate gland. The prostate is full of pleasure-potential for a man. You can access the prostate through the anus, which is why anal play for men can be so enjoyable. For a man, exploring his prostate may be a new experience for him, and he may be a little bit skeptical, especially since it involves the anus. Anal play can be for everyone and anyone, and it has the potential to make a man reach new levels of orgasmic pleasure. The prostate is a secret weapon of such intense pleasure that you would be doing your man a disservice if you did not help him explore it.

A man can begin to explore his prostate independently if he is not quite comfortable doing it with a partner. He can begin by including it in his next masturbation session to give himself a little extra love. Once he experiences the prostate sensations and feels comfortable and full of excitement about this newly discovered area of his body, he can also try it with a partner and show them how to please him in this way.

If this is something that you would like to try, you can first try to have an anal orgasm on your own during masturbation. Once you have done this, it will be much easier to take what you have learned into the bedroom with your partner and show them how best to touch you there. Once you have figured out the best way to pleasure yourself anally, this can be a fun and a very pleasing new addition to your sex life. If your partner knows how to touch you there, this can drive you crazy with pleasure. Below, I am going to share a few tips with you for anal sex. These tips will help both the man and the woman know to make the experience as smooth and pain-free as possible.

The anus is a very sensitive area for women, contrary to the beliefs of some people. While it is well-known that men have sensitive anuses and can receive pleasure here, it is a less well-known fact that so can women. Women have very sensitive anal openings because there are many nerve endings and a lot of surface area. This sensitivity means that when stimulated, a woman can feel a lot of pleasure here. Because this is an area that rarely receives a stimulation, it can be much more enjoyable for a woman because she may not have experienced these sensations before.

What the Kama Sutra Says About Anal Sex

The Kama Sutra mentions anal sex as one of the main forms of sex that can exist. It specifically says that anal sex can be practiced by heterosexual couples and homosexual couples, demonstrating the relevance of the Kama Sutra to this day.

The Lower Congress

As you now know, the Kama Sutra talks about sex in terms of "The Congress." When discussing anal sex, the Kama Sutra calls it *the lower congress.* Since anal sex encompasses anything sexual that you do to a person's anus, the Kama Sutra also discusses fingering and penetrative acts as sex types. For this reason, we will look at different types of anal sex in the following section.o

When talking about anal sex, the Kama Sutra says that a man and woman should emulate how animals have sex, as that is natural. This section will share a few different anal sex positions that you and your partner can try together to increase intimacy.

1. Reverse Cowgirl With Anal Play

The Reverse Cowgirl position is one included in the Kama Sutra section on traditional intercourse, but here we are going to learn about how you can use it for anal pleasure as well.

This position is a position that allows for the possibility of multiple female orgasms. Get into the reverse cowgirl position, which means that the man lies down on the bed on his back, and the woman straddles his penis. However, she is facing his feet instead of his head. The woman can grind her hips on the man's penis and control the penetration speed and depth from this position. However, to make it an advanced position, she will lean forward and grab onto his ankles for support. Then, he can begin to play with her anus using his fingers or a toy. He does not need to penetrate her there; necessarily, he can just play with the outside of her anus, and she will still feel immense pleasure.

If penetration occurs both anally and vaginally, though, she may have a blended orgasm in this way. She can have multiple back-to-back orgasms here if she has a vaginal orgasm. The man continues to stimulate her anal opening, which will keep her aroused and cause her to have another vaginal orgasm. This repeated orgasm could happen a few times over in a single session, as the anal play will keep her aroused and wanting more as she keeps having vaginal orgasms.

2. Rimming

Start by having your partner lie face down on the bed. Get behind them, straddle one of their legs and begin caressing and kissing their butt cheeks. You want to make them feel relaxed and comfortable for it to feel good for them. Continuing to massage and touch, slowly work your way closer to the middle. Start kissing their lower back and move lower, kissing the whole way down for a little tease. Spread their cheeks with your hands. With their cheeks spread, begin to gently move your tongue around their cheeks and the outside of their butthole. The key is to move slowly and gently to not reflexively tense up their butt cheeks and/or hole. Gently move your tongue around it in slow circles, and as they relax and settle into pleasure, you will be able to get in a little bit, and as it progresses, a bit deeper. Use your hands to massage their cheeks while you explore with your tongue, and every so often, you can use your finger to massage the hole as well. Continue in this way, moving inside and around, and listen as they moan in pleasure louder than you have ever heard before.

3. Doggy Style Anal Sex

This position is similar to the traditional Doggy Style position, where the woman is on all fours, and the man kneels behind her. Instead of penetrating her vaginally in this position, he will instead penetrate her anally. This position gives them both the opportunity to change the speed and depth of penetration, according to their feelings. A woman can also do this position to a man if she is wearing a strap-on dildo. This position is a great position for couples who are new to pegging, as the man and woman can adjust the position easily.

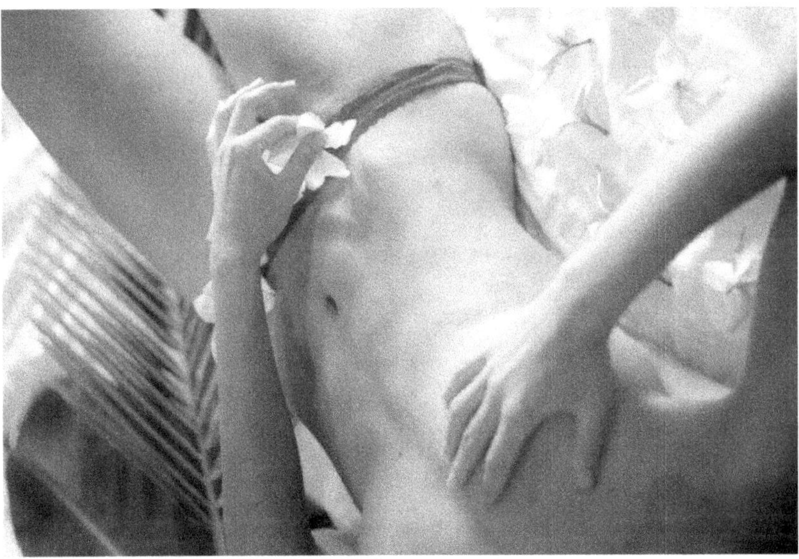

Before we move on, I want to give you some more advice to keep in mind when it comes to anal sex. Before beginning any sort of anal sex, there are some things which you should keep in mind. In this section, we will look at some tips for anal sex safety.

Firstly, anal sex requires a lot of lube since the anus cannot lubricate itself the same way that the vagina can. Next, if you will be using a toy for anal sex, make sure to wash it thoroughly afterward, *especially* before putting it into another hole like the vagina. Keeping this tip in mind will keep it clean and prevent the woman from getting a bladder infection. Third, when having anal sex, especially for the first time, you will need to take it slow. There is no need to rush. The key is to ensure the woman is comfortable with the depth and speed of penetration before going deeper or faster. The anus will relax and widen as you stimulate it more, so be patient.

The Kama Sutra Theories Of Relationships

There are a variety of different relationships that the Kama Sutra discusses. Some of these relationships happen between a woman and a married man, some are between a man and his mistress, and others involve group relationships. Below I have outlined some of the different relationships that the Kama Sutra talks about, including how the Kama Sutra says that these individuals should interact when it comes to sex.

Because love and sex do not work in a "one-size-fits-all" manner, there is a type of relationship out there that fits you personally the best! Being open with yourself and with your potential partner can help you to find this.

- Monogamous Relationships

Monogamous relationships are the relationships that people first learn about and likely think of. They are the most traditional out of all types of relationships and most often easiest for children to understand as they usually see this exhibited by their parents. The people who are in monogamous relationships have one single romantic partner or sexual partner at one time. Most people who enter monogamous relationships intend to remain monogamous, although it may not stay that way.

- Polyamorous Relationships

Some people choose to enter a relationship that is polyamorous instead. When a person identifies as polyamorous, it means that they are comfortable and have the desire to have more than one romantic relationship at the same time. Usually, within polyamorous couples, one or both persons will have a primary partner, a secondary partner, and so forth. They have an understanding that these 'rankings' are subject to change when their personal needs change. Some people in these relationships may treat every relationship that they have as perfectly equal. Like this book's theme, the key to any successful relationship, especially polyamorous ones, is effective and honest communication between everybody.

- Open Relationships

Open relationships are, in some ways, a blend between monogamous and polyamorous relationships. An open relationship allows both partners to have sexual relations with other people, but they reserve their emotional intimacy for each other only. Each person can have as many sexual partners as they want, but they will only have one romantic partner.

- Long-Distance Relationships

This type of relationship is pretty self-explanatory. A long-distance relationship occurs when both people have a large distance separating their physical presence. Since these relationships lack physical intimacy due to living far apart, some people opt for an open relationship while they are in different places. Although this relationship's 'long-distance' aspect is usually temporary, some couples choose and can have a happy relationship while living apart indefinitely.

- Casual Sex Relationships

When two people are in a casual sex relationship, they agree to have regular sex with each other, and that's pretty much in. Those in these types of relationships can be both physically and emotionally intimate with other people and long as both parties are comfortable. Casual sex relationships can also be 'exclusive,' which means that both people cannot sleep with others. This type is similar to a monogamous relationship minus the emotional connection.

- 'Friends With Benefits' Relationships

This relationship is also very similar to the casual sex relationship but with one important differentiator – a platonic and established friendship. Often, 'friends with benefits' relationships begin when two people with an established friendship have sex out of a mutual sexual attraction. Both people behave platonically outside of the sexual relationship. Usually, this type of relationship comes to an end when one person or both persons begin to date, other people.

- Asexual Relationships

Some people identify as asexual, which means that they don't experience sexual attraction or desire for other people. However, they still want to have a romantic relationship built on emotional intimacy. Although asexual people often choose to date other asexual people to create a purely asexual relationship, this is not always the case. When a person who is asexual begins a relationship with a sexual person, it can occur in a few different forms. The couple can decide to be entirely sexless, or the asexual partner can 'compromise' by engaging in sexual activity under certain agreed circumstances. The partners can also experiment in 'pseudo-sexual behavior' like cuddling or an arrangement that works for both parties.

A relationship means something different to every person, and it also feels and looks different to everyone. It is for this reason that there are so many different types of romantic relationships. No matter what kind of relationship you are looking for, all consensual relationships are valid. The important part is that you must be honest with yourself about what you are looking for to find the most compatible person. Finding this person will save you from the disappointment and unhealthy boundaries that can result when people have mismatched expectations of their relationship and, thus, a lack of compatibility.

All 4 of the types of love described earlier in this book can be found in different capacities in different types of relationships, making the Kama Sutra relevant today.

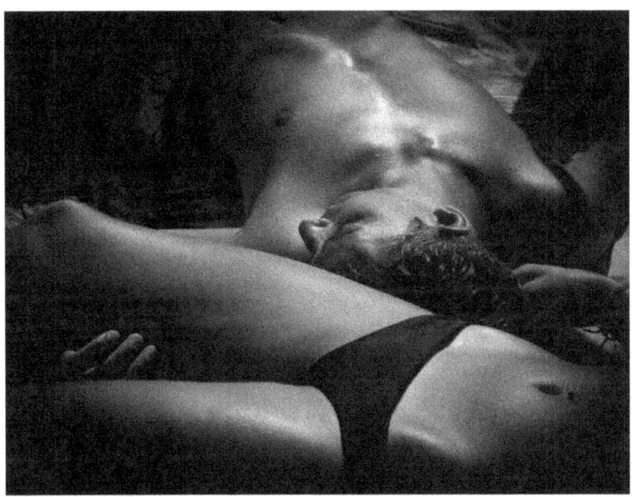

What the Kama Sutra Says About Group Sex

The previous section on relationships leads us here; our next topic is Group sex. Group sex may be a new concept to you, and it may seem like something that is only done in porn or talked about in certain circles of people. Still, there are many more people engaging in group sex than you may think. The Kama Sutra talks about group sex in various situations, which we will look at below. Before moving on, remember that the Kama Sutra discusses sex using the term *Congress*. You will see examples of this below.

The United Congress

The United Congress refers to a sexual encounter involving one man and two women. The Kama Sutra mentions that a man should enjoy sex with two women simultaneously, both of whom love him equally.

When a man is having sex with two women at once, this is called the *United Congress*.

The Congress Of The Herd Of Cows

The Kama Sutra also mentions group sex, though it may not be the type of group sex you would expect. The type of group sex that The Kama Sutra discusses involves many women and one single man.

When a man is enjoying sex with many women, this is called the *Congress of the Herd of Cows*.

The Gramaneri

Another form of group sex that The Kama Sutra discusses is something called *The Gramaneri*.

This kind of group sex involves many men that are having sex with one woman. The woman involved is usually married to one of the men present in this group sexual encounter. In this scenario, there are two options. The men could opt to have sex with the woman one at a time, each of the men taking a turn.

Alternatively, all of the men could have sex with the woman at the same time. For this option, the Kama Sutra specifies the following arrangement; One man holds the woman, another man penetrates her vaginally, another man is given oral sex by her, and another holds her "middle part." They will then alternate and continue to "enjoy her" in all areas, taking turns at each part of her body.

Keep in mind that Vatsyayana wrote The Kama Sutra long ago. He wrote it with the intention that men would read it, so he addressed it to them. Further, he wrote it in a time and place where a man could have multiple women simultaneously, even if he were married. It is for this reason that the section on group sex may seem dated or irrelevant today.

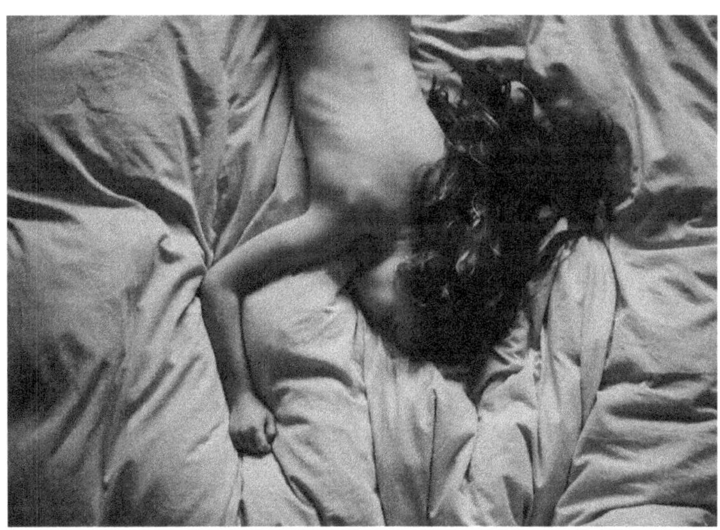

Sex Positions For These Situations

This section will look at several positions that will help you try group sex with your partner and anyone else you choose to include. These positions are a fun way to spice up your sex life by trying a new type of sexual experience.

Sexy Group Spin The Bottle

Before I begin explaining this position/activity, it is essential to note that each person taking part must provide consent before anyone else performs any sexual activity on them (or before they perform it on someone else). All parties involved must provide explicit verbal consent before they do any sexual act to someone else or before someone does any to them.

Traditional spin the bottle is done in a large group of people, with each person being an option the bottle can land on. Everyone sits in a circle with the bottle lying on its side in the middle. One person will spin the bottle on its side and whoever the bottleneck is facing when it stops spinning is the person that the spinner has to kiss.

In this sexy version of spin the bottle, I have changed some of the rules to make it sexier. While the basic rules are the same, there are a few more elements to it. This version is less of a sex position and more of a group sex activity. You can play this game with anything you have; all you'll need is some type of bottle, paper, and a pen. Think of a traditional spin, the bottle circle, with about five to ten people sitting in a circle.

There will also be a bowl or a basket with small pieces of paper in it, each with a different sexual act written on it. When the first person spins the bottle, the person it is pointing to when it stops spinning is the person who the spinner will need to perform the sexual act to (or with). The spinner will choose a piece of paper at random from the bowl after they spin, and this will determine which sexual act they must give. The group can decide which acts they want to write on the small slips of paper before they begin playing to ensure that everyone is comfortable.

This game serves as a great way to begin foreplay before engaging in penetrative group sex, as it can ease some nerves and get people acquainted with one another. Below, I have provided examples of sexual activities you can write on the slips of paper, but anything goes as long as you are all okay with it.

- Lick their nipples
- Please give them a hickey in a specific location
- Give them oral sex for 2 minutes, stopping before they reach orgasm
- Pick which position the two of you will engage in penetrative sex in after this game is over
- Please give them a lap dance

- Please give them a massage on a body part of their choosing for 2 minutes
- Take off their underwear using your mouth/teeth only
- Find the craziest sex position that you can find online, and you will attempt it together at some point in the encounter

Group Oral Sex Position

The first man lies down on his back on the bed, and the first woman straddles his face while he stimulates her genitals with his mouth and tongue. This position will be very good for the woman from a pleasure point of view because she can move her hips and grind herself on his face as she feels pleasure, to receive more pressure, or increase the speed by moving her hips. He can also use his hands to stimulate her clitoris, or he can grab onto her butt or slide a finger inside her vagina- all while he uses his mouth to please her clitoris. While this is happening, another person can do one of three things,

1. Stroke his penis using their hand while they are in this position so that he can feel physical pleasure as well
2. Suck on his penis with their mouth while also stimulating his testicles with their hands
3. Straddle him and have him penetrate them vaginally or anally with his penis

Finally, another man can stand in front of the first woman (who is straddling the man's face), and she can then stimulate his penis and testicles using her mouth and tongue.

In this position, they will all be able to reach orgasm somehow, as they are all giving and receiving pleasure. If anyone wishes, they can also stimulate their genitals using their hands or a sex toy such as a vibrator for maximum pleasure.

Depending on how many people are involved, more people can join by giving oral sex or penetrative sex to the other people already involved, making room for even more people.

How These Situations Will Improve Your Sex Life And Your Relationship

Trying new things in the bedroom with your partner will do nothing but great things for your relationship.

Archaeologists found evidence in drawings and sculptures dug up from ancient civilizations, which tells us a little bit about which sex positions people used long ago. One specific sculpture dates back to 9000 B.C., which is not the oldest visual evidence of sexual intercourse among humans. This sculpture shows two humans intertwined with one another in a sitting position, engaging in sexual intercourse. This position involves the man sitting down and the woman sitting on his lap, both of their arms and legs wrapped around one another in a tight embrace. They also discovered some drawings that depict Egyptians having sex in various positions, similar to the Doggy-Style position known and loved by many today. These depictions show chariots with women riding them, their buttocks in the air, and the man penetrating her from behind. They also show some variations of the Missionary position, where the man and woman are face to face, the man penetrating the woman from the front while she rests her leg on his shoulder. These positions are also known and loved by many these days.

While there is evidence of early sex positions such as these, it is in more modern days that they got labeled with names such as Doggy Style or Cowgirl. The modern-day also brings with it the introduction of sex toys and more adventurous positions involving acrobatics or more complex movements.

With all of this evidence, we are still unsure whether the difference here is that people are talking more about the interesting and new sexual positions they are trying or genuinely new and have come about as time has passed. The answer to this question may never become apparent. Still, this information serves as a reminder that humans have been having sex in various positions since the advent of time.

Just as animals do, humans rely on sex to keep the population growing. The advent of technology and changing cultures has led to more and more sex positions, sex toys, and sex-related technologies.

Chapter 7: More Ways to Improve

This chapter will help you become aware of some of the options available to you and your partner and how they can be used to maximize both male and female pleasure. After finishing this chapter, you will be aware of several new ways to spice things up in the bedroom with your partner.

Sex Toys

Sex toys may be something you are unfamiliar with, but they can bring fun, excitement, and new forms of pleasure to anybody's sex life. Sex toys increase and enhance your pleasure, contrary to popular belief; they are not for people who need help sexually or cannot perform well enough without them.

- The Cock Ring

The first toy we will look at is a cock ring. Originally, people used a cock ring to keep a man's penis hard for a longer time, though people use them for much more than that these days.

The cock ring was originally a ring made of metal and sat at the base of a man's penis to keep the blood inside the penis, which is responsible for causing an erection in the first place. These cock rings can be as tight as you want them to be, as they come in various sizes.

The cock ring will help the man last longer while also giving him the pleasure to have an erection for longer.

These days, you can get a cock ring that also has vibrating functions. This type of cock ring is great for couples. A cock ring like this works in much the same way as the original one, but we now make them out of a softer material like silicone, so it is a bit more comfortable for the man to wear. This type of cock ring begins vibrating with the push of a button or the flip of a switch.

While you wear this, it will not only keep you hard for longer, but it will also vibrate on the base of your penis. You can wear this while you are masturbating for added pleasure and endurance or while you are having sex with a partner for added endurance and pleasure for your penis. The bonus of wearing one of these while having penetrative sex with a partner is that the ring's vibration on your penis can also vibrate on the woman's clitoris. Because of a penis curve and the clitoris's position relative to the man's body in the missionary position, her clitoris could touch the penis' base during sex. Therefore she would also get the vibration of the ring. This positioning and clitoral vibration will give the woman a great orgasm!

This double pleasure works best in certain positions, like missionary, for example.

- The Dildo

A dildo is a penis-like object made of silicone that is to be inserted somewhere like the vagina or the anus. They can be beneficial for male and female pleasure, depending on how you use them. The world of dildos is vast and contains every kind of penetrative device you could dream of.

You can use a dildo with a partner as well as alone during masturbation.

If you like the feeling of the dildo, you can have your partner hold it and insert it into your vagina while you lie back and enjoy or while you massage your clitoris. Most dildos are waterproof, so you can take them into the bathtub or shower as well, so you can have some dildo shower sex if you wish.

You can use a dildo in the vagina or the anus, whichever you prefer, and you can use the same dildo for both of these places, so you don't need to buy two. If you want to use your dildo alone, you can insert it into your anus in a similar way as you should insert it into your vagina, or you can insert it into your vagina while you massage or penetrate your anus. You can do anything you like with a dildo and any combination of things.

There also exists a dildo that you can use for both male and female pleasure at the same time. This type is the double-ended dildo. Generally, you would not wear this dildo as a strap-on, but instead, you would insert it into the man's anus and either the woman's anus or her vagina. Then, both people can thrust towards each other to pleasure each other at the same time. This dildo can please the woman in multiple ways and please the man to a high degree anally.

While being penetrated in this way, the woman can also use a vibrator or other type of sex toy to stimulate her clitoris if she wishes.

The best position for exploring the maximum pleasure that this type of sex can achieve is when the man lies face-down on the bed, and the woman inserts the dildo into his anus slowly and with ample lube. The woman then positions herself face-down, but with her head at the opposite end of the bed from his. She slides the other end of the dildo into her vagina with her legs on either side of the man's body. She can then move her body up and down to slide the dildo in and out of her vagina. She can lift or lower herself using her arms to have the dildo enter her at different angles to have it hit her G-spot eventually. While she is doing this, it will also slide in and out of her partner's anus, stimulating his prostate and giving him great pleasure.

- The Vibrator

A vibrator is probably the most common sex toy available for female pleasure. Vibrators are the best choice for women who are new to sex toys and are unsure of what they may be looking for. A vibrator is a nice and easy place to start if you are new. Vibrators can be used in various ways- they can be used alone, during sex with a partner, or by a partner to you. You can use a vibrator during penetration and/ or foreplay.

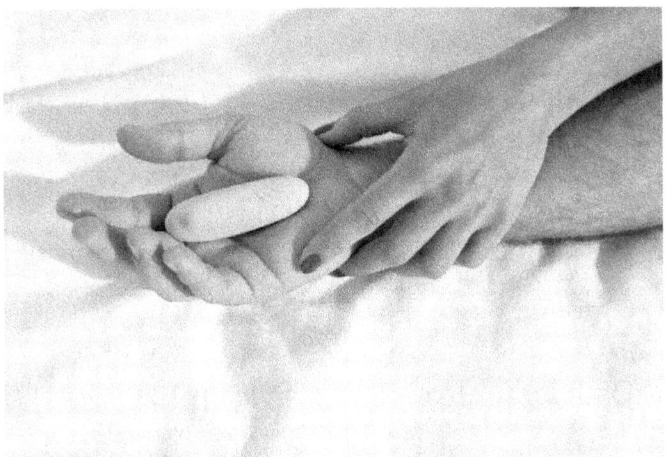

A Clitoral Vibrator

Vibrators are such a versatile sex toy, and they come in so many different shapes, sizes, and forms. The first type is called a *clitoral vibrator*. This type is small and compact, portable, and easy to use. You can activate this type with the push of a button. Once you

turn it on, you can hold it to your clitoris for quick and
intense clitoral pleasure in a way like nothing else.

Using a vibrator on the clitoris will give you great
pleasure because it can vibrate at speeds much higher
than a person's hands could ever reach. This level of
speed will be quite a new sensation, but one that you
won't soon forget and will be quite eager to have
again.

Some vibrators are slightly bigger than clitoral
vibrators and have a piece on them that you insert
into the vagina. These vibrators allow for both vaginal
penetration (so that you can stimulate your G-Spot) as
well as vibrating clitoral stimulation- so that you can
feel both of these types of pleasure at the same time!
This double sensation will be a new world of pleasure
for you as you may never have had both your clitoris
and your G-Spot stimulated at the same time. These
vibrators look like a phallic-shaped object usually
made of silicone that has a section partway down that
juts out in a small bump-like shape that is the part
that touches your clitoris. The entire vibrator will
vibrate so that you will also feel some of this vibration
on your G-Spot for maximum pleasure.

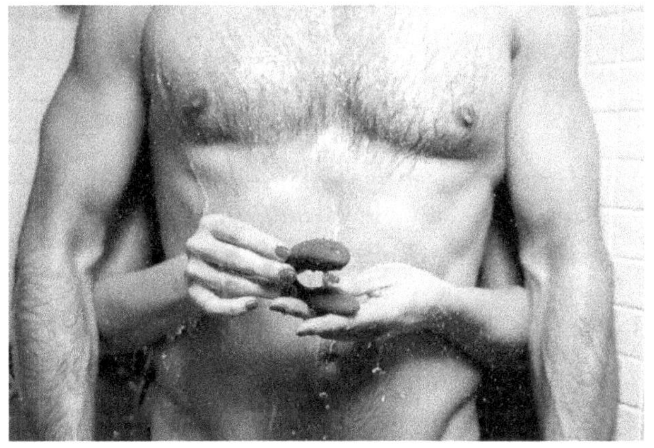

The next type of vibrator we will look at is a vibrating dildo. This kind of vibrator combines the dildo with the vibrator to give ultimate pleasure. This type is great for the woman and the man because he can feel the vibration on his penis if he penetrates the woman anally while she uses the dildo on herself.

- The Butt Plug

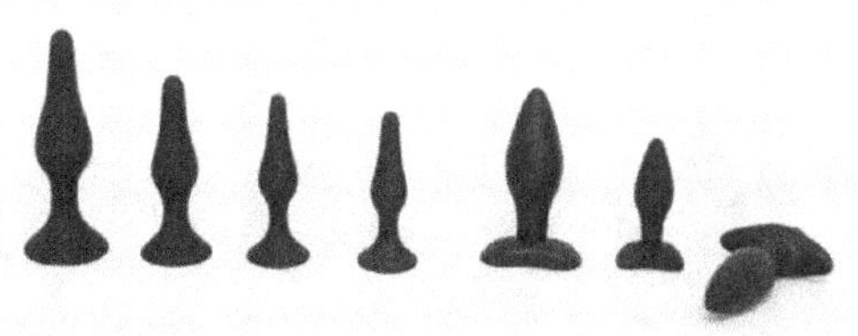

A butt plug is a small plug-type device that is inserted into the anus and is left there. This anal sex toy gives a person pleasure because of the stretching of the anal opening, which, as I mentioned, is very sensitive. It also provides a person with pleasure because of the stretching of the entire anal canal in general.

The butt plug is a toy that you can use passively to give you pleasure while you are doing other things like penetrative vaginal sex or oral sex. As you move, you will feel pleasure from the pressure it puts on the inside of your anus. This sex toy can be used by either a man or a woman while engaging in other sexual activities with a partner or alone during masturbation. Some people like to insert their butt plug to get them in the mood for sex before their clothes even come off!

Role-Playing

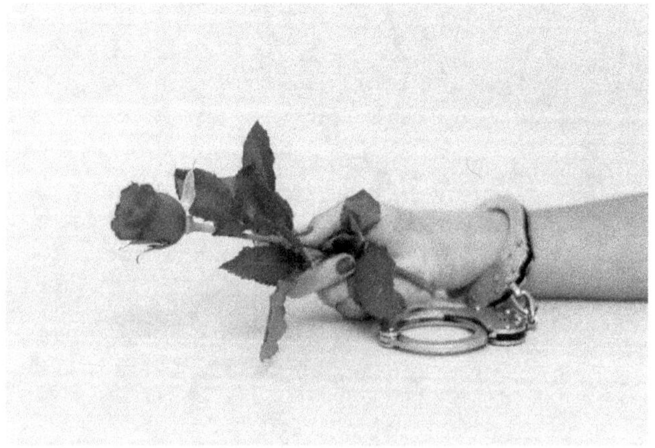

Role Play can be an enjoyable and really hot way to get out of your head and into your body. You can try different role-playing scenarios that turn you on or act out fantasies you have. It gives you a way to explore different characters and roles that may turn you on in the movies or porn.

A role play usually includes a dominant person (dom.) and a submissive person (sub.). There is usually one character in a role play with more power (teacher, boss) over the other (student, secretary). This kind of sexual encounter is where the concept of *Dom* and *Sub* comes in.

One partner will play the dominant role, and the other will play the submissive role in a role play, which will add to your pleasure because the dominant character may 'punish' or scold the submissive partner.

Most people become very turned on by being in one of these two roles. To find out if you get turned on by being dominant or submissive in your sex life, play around with both sides and see which one makes you hot for more and makes you feel like you are acting in a bad play. Everyone's role play preferences will be different, but we will explore the *office romance* role play as an example.

Go into your office at home if you have one or if not, the dining room will work as well. Sit down at the table as if you are working in your office. You can set up this role-play together by planning ahead, or you can start it spontaneously. If you begin spontaneously, your partner can play along when they realize what you are getting at. Your woman will then come in and greet you formally, saying something like, "Hey, I reviewed this document and had a few questions." Continue the role play and let your fantasies come to life. To transition it to a sexy encounter, begin making out and imagine that you are in an office, so there is the possibility of being found out. This element of fear will bring a sexy thrill to your role play.

You can have sex while leaving some clothes on to emulate the scenario of needing to leave clothes on in case you need to quickly 'get back to work' will make this feel even more real. Have your woman lean forward over the desk and lift her skirt. Pull her panties down just enough, take your penis out of your trousers just enough, and enter her from behind. At any moment, you may need to pretend like nothing was happening, say if your boss knocks on your office door. Let yourselves get really into this role play, and you both will get so turned on by the different roles you get to play, you will be thinking of what role play to try next.

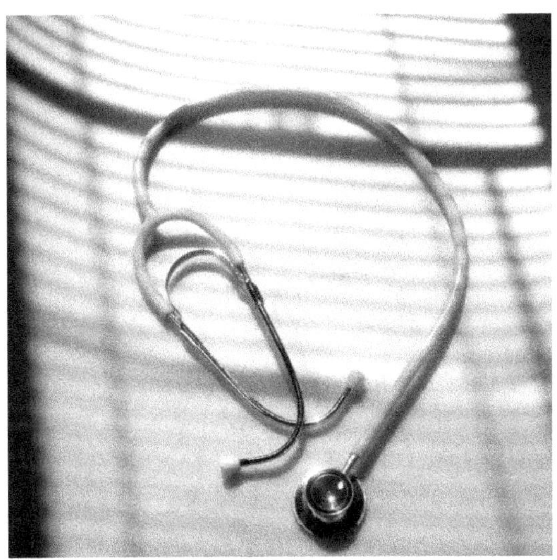

Some other common examples of role-playing include the following;

- Nurse and patient
- Student and teacher
- A police officer and a criminal
- Plumber and housewife
- Pizza delivery person and homeowner
- Masseuse and client

You are now aware of some ways that you can spice up your sex life with your partner, but here we will look at a few more before ending this chapter.

Everyone has sexual acts or themes that turn them on, but you must get in touch with this part of yourself to find out what your own are. In this section, we will look at how you can discover your sexual fantasies and fetishes.

First, though, we will look at some specific sexual fantasies to get an idea of what you are looking to discover. Under the umbrella of sexual fantasies is included the following, among others;

- Roleplay

If your sexual fantasy or kink is role play, you likely become aroused when you imagine playing a certain role in the bedroom with your partner like a homeowner, and he is a plumber coming to fix your pipes.

- Domination and Submission

If your kink or fetish is domination and submission, you likely become turned on by playing a certain role in bed- either being dominated by your partner or being dominant over them.

- Specific Sexual Acts

Your kink could also be something that is a specific sexual act. These can include spanking, hair pulling, or Piss Play.

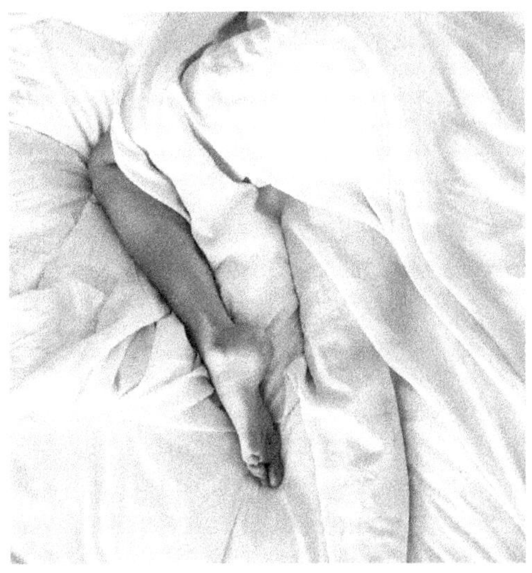

There are so many things that you can include in these categories to get yourself, and your partner turned on. There are so many more categories of their own. Many categories will overlap and cross over each other. For example, a police and convict role play fantasy could cross over into domination and submission play as well. By getting an idea of what is out there, you can begin to explore what you like the idea of and what you don't like sexually.

Conclusion

Thank you for reaching the end of this book; I hope it was full of useful information! I want to leave you with one final piece of advice, which we will look at below.

How To Talk To Your Partner About Sex

Now that you have finished reading this book, you may be wondering how you can begin to incorporate this new knowledge into your sex life. The first step to doing this is to talk to your partner about what you have learned. Sex is a two-way street, so you will need to get them on board with you.

Sometimes in a long-term relationship, you become so comfortable that you don't have to communicate as much as you used to since you know each other so well. The key here is to continue communicating, even if you think the other person knows what you are thinking or feeling without you having to say it. By doing this, you keep the lines of communication open in your relationship and avoid any chance of miscommunication or misunderstanding that would be perpetuated by a lack of communication. Having misunderstandings go unresolved could lead to resentment and an overall breakdown in communication, reducing the relationship's intimacy levels.

Remember our discussion of intimacy earlier on in this book. This intimacy and vulnerability include communicating about your desires- be they sexual desires or any other sort of desires. By sharing these thoughts and desires with your partner, you will be able to ensure that they know how to please you in every sense of the word. This discussion also leads to boundaries being set and upheld since your desires include things you are comfortable and okay with, and this conversation will often lead to things you are not okay with.

By learning these things about your partner, you can begin to work together to ensure each person meets the other's intimacy needs. For example, suppose your number one intimacy preference is for emotional intimacy, and your partner likes to show their love in physical ways. In that case, you can discuss how they can begin to be more vocal about their love for you, and you can be more receptive to their physical displays of affection. Putting these things out on the table for discussion is the best way to learn about each other. You can never stop learning about your partner, and this will only strengthen your relationship.

How To Open Up The Dialogue

Below, I have provided you with some steps for doing this with your partner.

Many people feel stagnant or that their sex life has become dull. It is natural to feel this way in a long-term relationship or have simply been having casual sex for quite some time and seek a deeper connection. This section will look at how you can get out of this sexual rut in a few simple steps. Keep in mind that these steps are simple, but putting them into practice will take some work and some effort on your part and your partner's part as well.

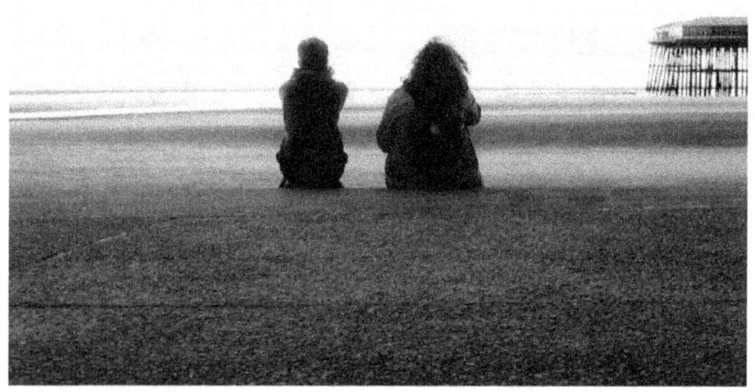

Step 1: Reach deep within yourself to find what it is that you need and what it is that you want from your sex life as well as in terms of pleasure.

Step 2: Take some time to explore this within yourself and find out more about it. Be curious about yourself.

Step 3: Communicate this to your partner in an open and honestly vulnerable way. This communication can be with your sexual partner or with your romantic partner- whoever you will be having sex with and sharing this with.

Step 4: Put this into practice by maintaining communication with your partner and exploring it with them.

Step 5: Ask your partner to communicate back to you. Ask them to communicate about what they want and need after giving them some time to reach deep within themselves to find out what they want and need.

Step 3 and Step 5 are often points of confusion or distress for many people, as they may not know where to begin when approaching this type of conversation. Below, I have given you several ways to initiate this type of conversation and things that you can ask your partner to help them open up about these things if they have some trouble doing so.

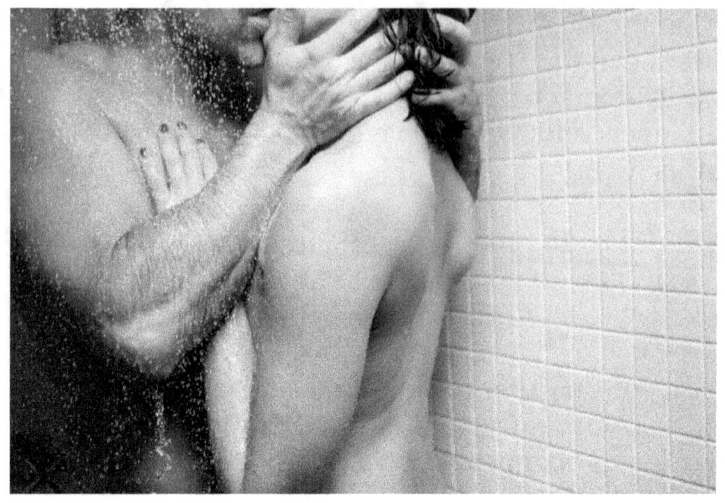

To begin with, this type of conversation will require honest self-expression. Honest self-expression means expressing oneself authentically in a way that is likely to inspire compassion in others. Expressing your true feelings and ensuring that the feelings you are expressing are the deepest ones you could find is quite intimidating and can make you feel extremely vulnerable. Connecting this deep feeling to a need is also another stage of vulnerability. Sharing your needs and values is likely not something that you often do. By sharing these things at one time is sure to make you feel very vulnerable. These two things are both ways of expressing yourself authentically. Therefore, you are practicing honest self-expression. By deciding to be vulnerable even though it is hard and uncomfortable, this inspires compassion in others. This vulnerability happens because they can see you deciding to be vulnerable and open with them about your feelings. Everyone can relate to how difficult this is, which makes them feel empathy or compassion for you in this situation. Second, because you are expressing a need and know that this is a difficult thing to do, they will also feel empathy or compassion for this need, as being vulnerable shows them that this is important to you.

From this honest self-expression, you can then begin to speak up about your deep feelings, including your wants and needs in a sexual sense. Once you do so, and you would like to encourage your partner to do the same. You can do this by having a deep and open conversation with them about sex. You can do this by using the questions below to help you start the conversation.

What they do and don't like:
In terms of sex acts, this could be anything like oral sex, fingering, anal, and other butt stuff or anything they enjoy, no matter how big or small. These could be things they have tried before, want to try in the future, have never tried before, or that they know they do not want to try. Keep this question very open-ended to get the maximum amount of information possible.

What she needs and likes during foreplay specifically:
This point is more pertinent to a woman, but you can ask this of a man. This point could include the length of time she needs, what acts she likes done to her, and what she likes to do to you during foreplay if she likes

kissing to be included or not and what it takes to get her into the mood and wet enough for penetration.

Specifically, what they like and don't like that you do or have done:
These are things specifically related to the two of you having sex with each other. The other questions in this list can include anything in their past or anything they have not yet tried. This question in particular, though, involves only the two of you and your sex life together. Try not to take it too personally if they tell you there is something they do not enjoy as much as you thought they did. This conversation is all about growth and learning.

What, if anything, makes them orgasm almost instantly:
Maybe something they do for themselves during masturbation or something they know will set them off instantly in the best way. This answer could be something you do for them or something they like to do to themselves.

What their favorite positions are:
This question involves asking them about their favorite sex positions, both for penetrative sex and for sex not involving penetration. What they like about these positions would also be beneficial for you to know.

Any kinks or fetishes they may have:
Both that they have experience with and that they may be just discovering for the first time. If your partner is

unsure, ask them if they are open to exploring new kinks with you. Maybe you both will find new things that you enjoy.

Anything they have wanted to do sexually specifically with you:
Maybe you have never done a 69 together, but they enjoy this position, or maybe they saw something in a porn video that they would like to try. Maybe there is something that your partner has wanted to experiment with, and they are wondering if you would be open to it.

Anything they have been fantasizing about trying:
Maybe a role-play or a specific location, maybe a fantasy that they are embarrassed to talk about. This question is last on the list because hopefully, at this point, the conversation is flowing a little easier, and your partner will be more comfortable answering this question by now. Make your partner feel comfortable and let them know that anything they disclose to you will remain between you and your partner.

While these questions are extremely personal, you can make them feel comfortable being open about these topics. This conversation will require a lot of vulnerability on both of your parts, so showing them that you are listening intently and assuring them that you are doing so without judgment is important. Suppose they seem very hesitant to open up about these things- and they might, depending on the age of your relationship and their level of openness about sex in general. In that case, you can ask them if they would rather you answer these same questions first, and they can answer them afterward. This conversation may make them feel less like they are on the spot and more comfortable with the conversation as a mutual exchange.

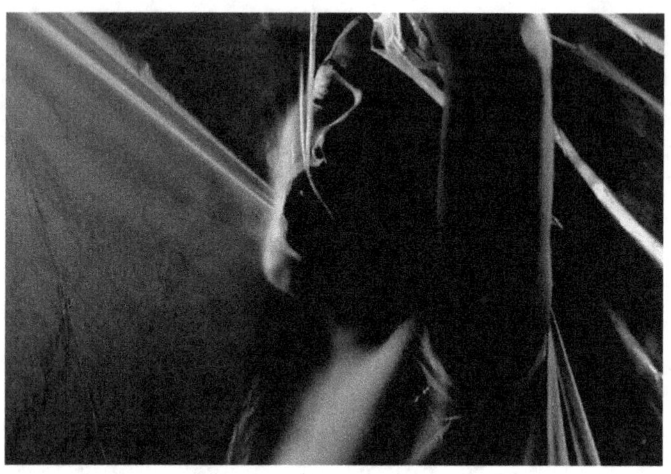

I hope that you are leaving this book, having learned a few new things to take with you into your sexual adventures from here forward. I hope this serves as a tool for you to explore and discover yourself and your future partners. The main focus was to share strategies for maintaining a deep emotional connection with your long-term partner and teach you how to accomplish this through sex. Contained within was an abundance of tips and suggestions on exactly how to continue to have an intimate and loving marriage or relationship for years to come from the Kama Sutra's perspective.

As you continue your relationship with your partner, you never know when the knowledge this book has bestowed on, you will prove useful. You may want to try something new on an anniversary getaway and think of the perfect position to try. You may be having a discussion with your friends about marriage and sex. You may think of how you learned that intimacy must be maintained and worked at to remain strong. This knowledge will remain in the back of your mind until the time you need it most, and then it will pop to the front of your mind to help yourself, your partner, or your friends. You can never be too knowledgeable about sex and relationships. By taking the step to read this book in its entirety, you are only helping yourself out for the rest of your life- your sex life, your romantic life, and your life in general.

If you like this book, please leave a review on Amazon so that others can discover and benefit from this book just like you!